Shadow On My Soul:

Overcoming Addiction to Suicide

By Paula M. Quinn, Ph. D.

Cover Design: Gil Fahey
Text Design: Robin McArdle

Library of Congress Cataloging in Publication Data

Quinn, Paula M.
    Shadow on my soul: overcoming an addiction to suicide / by Paula
M. Quinn.
      p.   cm.
    ISBN 1-879198-13-4 (paper)
    1. Quinn, Paula M. 2. Adult child abuse victims--United
States--Biography. 3. Depressed persons--United States--Biography.
4. Suicidal behavior--Case studies. 5. Healing--Case studies. I. Title.
RC569.5.C55Q56   1995
616.85'8445'0092--dc20
   [B]   95-3883
                                                  CIP

First Published in 1995 by:
Knowledge, Ideas & Trends, Inc.
1131-0 Tolland Turnpike, Suite 175
Manchester, CT 06040
Telephone: 1-800-826-0529

ISBN 1-879198-13-4

10 9 8 7 6 5 4 3 2 1

Printed in the United States of America

The author urges those who suffer from depression and suicidal thoughts to seek professional help through local mental health agencies, from local medical professionals, or by calling the following toll-free numbers where sincere, compassionate and confidential assistance is available 24-hours a day:

Suicide Crisis and Referral Service: 1-800-877-7675
Suicide Prevention Helpline: 1-800-333-4444

Darkling I listen;
and for many a time I have been
half in love with easeful Death.
Called him soft names in many a mused rhyme,
to take into the air my quiet breath;
now more than ever seems it rich to die...

from Ode to a Nightingale by John Keats

Table of Contents

I would like to pay special tribute to Dr. Pat Carr of the Department of English at Western Kentucky University, whose inspiring words, "to tell our stories on behalf of those who have similar stories to tell, yet who cannot write," gave me the courage to begin writing this book, and whose generosity of time and talent enabled me to complete it.

And to Dr. Ward Hellstrom, former Dean of Potter College of Arts and Sciences at Western Kentucky University, who believed enough in me, in my story, and in what it might mean to others, that he gave me the opportunity, the time, and above all, the encouragement to write this book, and in so doing, helped me to discover a crucial lesson: that when you have healed, you share what you have learned.

Acknowledgements

I would like to thank the following people in the order in which they came into my life, just when I needed them:

My son, Ivan Miner Quinn and my daughter, Claire Jena Quinn, who have given to their mother unconditional love, understanding and friendship; Sandra Horn, who talked me into buying my first computer; Terry Weis Langford, who encouraged me to follow my own path; members of the mediation group who encouraged me in spiritual development and holistic health; administrators, faculty and staff of Western Kentucky University including Jo-Ann Albers, chairman, Department of Journalism, and Jim Highland, print journalism sequence coordinator, Dr. David Lee, Dean of Potter College of Arts, Humanities and Social Sciences and Dr. Robert Haynes, Vice President for Academic Affairs, all of whom approved valuable faculty release time for me; Suzie Hardin and Voletta Havener, the journalism department's supportive secretaries; and WKU's wonderfully helpful librarians; Mike Arduser, who suggested the organization of the chapters; Hannelore Hahn and the members of the International Women's Writing Guild for their loving encouragement; and my expert editor, Rita McCullough.

Finally, my deepest gratitude to the hundreds of students I have taught through the years: Your love and interest in me both as your teacher and as your friend, helped save my life. You are truly angels unaware.

For my children
and
for the Earth:
Provider, comforter, teacher, healer.

Shadow On My Soul:

Overcoming Addiction to Suicide

By Paula M. Quinn, Ph. D.

Chapter 1

Depression

This is the feeling that comes over me every fall: acute depression characterized by hopelessness; a chest so heavy I cannot draw breath; burning eyes, sad eyes, empty eyes, mirrors of my insides, eyes whose lids feel so heavy I have difficulty looking up.

Sometimes I think it's my mascara so I change brands or buy a new tube; but no, that's not it. Sometimes I think it's my contact lenses and I put them away for a week or two; but no, that's not it. Sometimes I think it's food, that if I eat nothing but plain yogurt and unsalted, unsweetened bread, and fruits and vegetables, then I will feel well again, have hope, smile and mean it, be glad; but no, that's not it either. I am still deeply depressed, still drawing breaths that are erratic and heavy, still filled with this enormous weightiness that touches every fiber of my body.

I pray. I meditate. I think positive, happy thoughts. I try to keep all negativity--people, places, things--from me. I review the day and see that, from an intellectual point of view, it has been yet another good one. But still, the heaviness, the hopelessness, the desire to curl up as a fetus and sleep and sleep is overwhelming.

I run, trying to add an extra city block each morning. I walk to my office once, twice--as many as four times a day-- but still, the depression is with me, engulfing me, stealing my soul.

I look for others to help, thinking that in so doing, I will take away my indefatigable ego, thereby making Self and Depression disappear. No luck there, either.

Once, when I was 14 or 15, I wrote a poem about a tiger. I think it was William Blake's "Tyger, Tyger" that inspired me to write about my own beast. I remember clearly the night eyes, the savage claws, and the line, "Stalking, stalking, stalking--ME!"

How often those words come back to me when I am severely depressed! I don't have to turn, to look over my shoulder or behind me--I know the tiger is there, savage, brutal, waiting to strike. The question is when-- and how.

This one thought bedevils me--the how. If I kept a gun, I would be dead right now, another number in the senseless census of lost lives. The desire to kill myself happens suddenly, in one of those devastating moments when all the hatred and anger and whatever frustration has been festering that particular time suddenly surges upward in a grand and powerful stroke, up through my genitals, through my chest, behind my face and up, into my brain in one enormous, overwhelming, physical shift. Surely something physiological is taking place, but at that moment, the physical doesn't enter into it. What matters most is the thought that comes instantly, automatically: "I'll just kill myself." And the tiger suddenly reclines.

Strange, isn't it, that that one simple thought, that one simple sentence could give such release. But it does. Why? Because it's an out, an escape, and yes, a solution. It's the solution I have been fighting all of my life: this impulse to self-destruct collides with the impulse to live.

How did I get this way this time? I try to think back, rationally, to late August, to early September. Ah, yes. Several days before the Labor Day weekend I began feeling exhausted and angry. For me, the two go hand in hand. If I'm too tired after work to do laundry and cook and clean, the work begins to build. What was something small, like a hill that I could climb suddenly erupts like Vesuvius all around me. I become resentful if I cannot do it all.

Well, I reasoned with myself, you should be drained. School has started and you teach four writing courses--a heavy load! You're going to bed late and getting up early to run with the dog so both of you will get some exercise. You're a single parent; you must do it all--feed and clothe two teenagers--pay all the bills, work with your students. This is how I reasoned with myself. Once again, it didn't work.

There are other symptoms of my depression. I feel scattered, unfocused, unproductive. I become clumsy and awkward, a disoriented bumbler who often stumbles and drops things. I struggle to think clearly and am almost constantly beset by a confusion of thoughts. I stutter and mispronounce words, or the precise word or phrase simply won't come. I can't remember how to spell. In grading a paper, I couldn't spell Kentucky--the place where I live! The sheer exhaustion, woven together with these other emotions drape themselves around me as an invisible shroud.

"Maybe you're getting sick. There's some kind of flu going around again." Was it my son or my daughter who said it this time? Why can I never say this myself, never think to myself, "I must be getting sick." I don't know that I have ever had this thought. Is it because I haven't learned to take care of myself, haven't learned to put me to bed, haven't learned that it's okay to lie down, to sleep when I'm unwell?

I love the word, the notion, caretaker. The thought transports me to my beloved Manitoulin Island in Canada where I see myself, a solitary figure, tending the wildflowers in the forests and fields along Lake Huron. But I can take care of myself about as much as I, alone, would be able to tend all of those acres.

Labor Day weekend the three of us had a crashing flu--sore throats, aches, fever, the works. We called ourselves bums because we didn't shower but lay around, reading, watching baseball games on television, resting. And then it was back to school on Tuesday.

I didn't feel much better, but I went back to classes anyway because I didn't want to get behind and I thought I would spend far less time feeling miserable if I kept busy. I was right, and wrong. What I didn't realize is that while my physical symptoms seemed to dissipate, the emotional feelings related to the illness were lurking somewhere around me, waiting to spring.

A key characteristic of my depression at these times is overwhelming anger that is hard to keep at bay. I am able to contain it until I walk in the house, then there it is, the snarling beast within, yelling at the kids, browbeating them, telling them how tough my life is, how I can no longer keep up with things, how I wish I were dead.

Their response is always the same: they automatically scramble into action, setting the table, sweeping the floor, shoving laundry into the washer, vacuuming the rugs--like two whirling dervishes who wish with all their young hearts that when they've finished reeling at my words, everything will be okay again. My behavior has taught my kids to be "fixers"--make it better and we'll have Mama an extra day.

What is their anodyne? Is it helping with supper? Emptying the wastebaskets? Feeding the pets? Try as they might, Ivan and Claire have not found the solution to our particular dysfunction. The result is their own frustration, worry and guilt, shortened attention spans at school, broken hearts at bedtime.

Here is a scene that illustrates better than I can tell what it is like to be so swept away by conflicting emotions that I wish I were dead. Ivan has a good friend, Jeff Gerard, who sometimes stays overnight. This particular weekend Jeff stayed two nights--he had my permission to do so. But by the evening of the second day I was so tired of cooking for kids, driving kids, talking to kids, that I went into one of my rages. Ivan and Jeff got into a little argument while playing a computer game. Jeff went upstairs. Ivan complained to me that our home was boring, and I went berserk. The last, among many things that I said to him, was, "I just wish I were dead."

It was dark in the dining room when I said this to my son. Moments later, as Jeff passed through on his way to the bathroom, Ivan drew back his fist in the darkness and hit Jeff, hard, in the jaw. If ever there was misplaced, misdirected anger, it came out that night, in my son.

Ironically, sadly, both Ivan and Jeff had become victims of my displaced rage.

Chapter 2

Chedge

"Mother! Mother, guess what!"

Sharon and I shouted excitedly as we bumped down the narrow hallway, each holding half of a bed pillow with a small red and white bear on top.

"What? What is it, girls? My! You sound so excited! Your mom's in here."

Aunt Jen and Mother were clearing the Sunday dinner dishes from the dining room table. Remnants of homemade chicken paprikash were glued to the plates and the table was strewn with crumbs from the pink cinnamon heart cake my Mother always made for my birthday. On this, my seventh, I had been able to choose the guests--Mother's youngest sister, Jen, Uncle Bill, who always called me "Sunshine" and their daughter, Pam, who, at 10, was like another sister to me and Sharon.

"Guess what, Mother?"

We waited for her to reply.

"What?"

"Pam said we could keep Chedge until the next time we got together!"

"That's Pam's bear, isn't it? You each got a nice Steiff bear from Germany for Christmas. You don't need another bear."

Sharon picked Chedge off his makeshift sedan chair and hugged him.

"But we love Chedge. He's so soft and cuddly. And our bears are all hard, like cement," Sharon said. "We can't dress them in doll clothes, either. They're too big. But Chedge is just the right size!"

"Yeah, Mama," I added. "And ours look mean. But Chedge is a nice bear. See? He's smiling."

As Sharon held Chedge up, her fingers made an impression in the bear's plump, dirty white velour tummy. She smoothed his floppy red ears and long red muzzle.

"Are you girls sure that's a bear?" Uncle Bill was leaning over the table, scooping some mixed nuts from the party dish. "He looks more like a mouse to me."

"Or a rat," Mother said.

"No, he's a bear, a wonderful, soft, cuddly little bear. Isn't he cute?" I said. I grabbed the bear away from Sharon and snuggled him under my chin.

"Hey! I was holding him! Wasn't I holding Chedge, Mother? Tell Paula to give him back!"

"But it's my turn. I want to hold Chedge. Besides, it's my birthday, so I get to hold him now."

"But you're not to grab things away from your sister! Now give that thing back to her."

I started to cry.

"Go, on! And if you don't stop crying, Pam will have to take him home. Maybe you should anyway, Pam. The way these two fight over things, there might be no Chedge left by the next visit.

"Where did you get him, anyway?"

Uncle Bill held up one finger--wait--while he chewed a mouthful of peanuts.

"I won him for Pam last summer at a carnival. It took me three baseballs to do it, but she got her bear." Uncle Bill smiled down at the daughter who had inherited his dark hair and almond-shaped brown eyes. "And you've slept with him every night since, haven't you, honey?"

Pam smiled and nodded.

"Well, I'm real proud of you for being willing to share him with Sharon and Paula. I think that's real nice of you."

I handed Chedge back to Sharon.

"Here, you can hold him for awhile. I'm sorry I grabbed him from you."

Mother began clearing more dishes from the table.

"If you take that thing from Pam, you'd better let her borrow something in return," Mother said.

"You can take Bruin."

"Yeah." I followed Sharon's lead. "And you can take Mr. Mole home, too. They've been together since Santa brought them for us. They're boyfriends."

"No they're not," Aunt Jen joked, "they're bearfriends."

We all laughed.

"Jen, why don't you and Bill and Pam go in by the fire in the living room and relax. I'll be in just as soon as the girls and I finish cleaning up. Then we can find Paul and play some cards, the four of us."

"Why don't Pam and I help, too? You've worked so hard cooking, the least we can do is help clean up."

"No, no. Go on, now, go relax. We know where everything belongs. It won't take more than a few minutes. Sharon, put the milk and butter away. Paula, pick up all the dirty silverware. We'll wash that first, before we do the dishes."

Sharon sat Chedge down carefully on the host's chair and tucked a birthday napkin over his chest and legs. She picked up the cranberry glass pitcher and butter plate and carried them into the kitchen. The door swung shut behind her.

"SSSS! SSSST!"

When we turned, Mother beckoned to us.

"What?" we whispered loudly in unison.

"Shh! Those bears are not leaving this house!"

She looked angrily from one of us to the other.

"You going to trade some ratty-looking piece of carnival junk for those two Steiff bears? Over my dead body!"

"He's not junk!" There were tears in Sharon's eyes.

"Well, I say he is junk! They didn't pay no thirty dollars apiece for that thing like I did for your two bears. Find something else for her to take home if you still want to trade."

"But Mother," I protested," we promised. We said Pam could take Bruin and Mr. Mole. What will we tell her if she can't?"

"I have no idea. That's your problem. But those bears are not leaving this house. And don't tell her I said so. Now dry your tears and get busy on these dishes."

Suddenly the door swung open and Aunt Jen came in. When she saw that Sharon had been crying, she picked up a party napkin, dried Sharon's tears, gave her a hug and told us to go and play.

Sharon went out one door and down the hallway to our bedroom where Pam was playing while I went out the other door to the dining room where Chedge was still sitting on the chair, his brown glass eyes staring at my half-eaten birthday cake. I scooped him up, gave him a kiss, and carried him past the kitchen on my shoulder.

"Ann," I could hear my aunt saying, "those bears of Sharon's and Paula's are just too nice for Pam to take home. I told her to pick out something else to keep for awhile."

"Really, Jen? Why? She can take them if she wants to."

"No, I don't think it would be a good idea," Aunt Jen said.

"If something happened to them, your kids would be heartbroken, especially Paula. I know how attached she gets to her dolls and stuffed animals, with that big heart of hers. No, Pam can find something else."

When they left around eight o'clock, Pam was carrying the two books she had borrowed. Sharon and I stood side by side in the doorway, each making Chedge wave good-bye with his paws.

"Thank you, Pam! We love you! Thanks for sharing! We'll take good care of Chedge," we called and called.

For the next month, our lives revolved around Chedge. We powdered him, diapered him, penciled eyebrows on him, dressed him, gave him rides in the doll buggy and held tea parties in his honor, took turns sleeping with him and fought over him.

On Good Friday there was no school, so Sharon and I were playing a quiet game of Uncle Wiggly in our bedroom. The bear sat propped on a pillow between us, and we were taking turns drawing cards for him. Chedge was winning. Suddenly, a sound came up through the heat register, a sort of scraping, and then groans.

We looked at each other, screamed and jumped up, yelling for our mother, who was doing laundry in the basement.

"Mother! Mother! There's a sound like a monster," Sharon yelled as we raced through the kitchen.

"Sharon! Chedge!"

I had suddenly realized that in our fright, we'd left the bear behind. I ran back to get him, then clattered down the stairs behind my sister, still yelling for our mother.

We passed the area with the clotheslines, and when we did not see Mother in the laundry room, tore to the rear of the basement, into the furnace room. She was not there, either.

Suddenly, we heard the noise again, but louder, a deep, rough sound echoing in the furnace. We screamed, turned around, and ran through the rooms calling for our mother. She was there, by the clotheslines, bent nearly double in laughter at our fright.

"You kids!" She lifted a corner of her apron to her eye. "You kids! Always afraid of everything! What is it this time?"

"A noise," Sharon said, "sort of a scraping, scratching sound. We heard that upstairs, and the roar, too, didn't we Paula?"

I cradled Chedge and shivering, looked around.

Mother listened intently.

"What do you mean? That?"

We nodded and drew closer to her. She looked deep into our faces.

"It's a monster in the furnace room."

I squealed and Sharon began to cry.

"Not," Mother said, laughing. "Not."

"How could you scare us like that?" Sharon asked.

Mother snorted.

"Scare you like what? I was just having a little fun. Besides, I was trying to get your attention. I want you to bring the wastebaskets down and empty them. Paula, you go while I calm down your sister."

I shook my head, no.

"What do you mean, no? I told you to do something."

I hugged Chedge tighter.

"I'm scared. I don't want to go up there alone."

I moved close to Sharon.

"Well, then go together. But go! I have enough to do already without having to do all the little chores, too. Come on, hurry up! And leave that dirty, motheaten bear down here. I'm so sick of seeing that filthy thing, I could scream. Now, move!"

We ran upstairs, combined the waste from three baskets into two, and were back downstairs in record time. We set the baskets at our mother's feet.

"Where's Chedge?" Sharon asked immediately. She peered behind the wet laundry on the lines.

"He's over there, on the bookshelf," Mother said. "You can have him as soon as you empty the baskets into the incinerator."

Neither of us moved.

"Now, what?"

"You come with us."

"What? Are you crazy? What for?"

"We're scared. We're scared to go back there, because of the noise, aren't we, Paula?"

I nodded.

"Eh, you're crazy. That was the furnace heating up that made those sounds. There's nothing back there. Now go."

Still, we didn't move. "All right then, I'll make you do as I say!" Mother shouted. She grabbed Chedge by one leg and stalked to the furnace room. Sharon and I each took a wastebasket and ran after her.

"Mother, we're sorry! We'll be good, we promise!" Sharon cried. "Please don't hurt Chedge!"

Mother stood behind the incinerator in the shadow of the furnace. Her arms were behind her back.

"Here are the baskets, Mother, please let us have Chedge!" Sharon was crying harder now.

I looked up at my mother's face. Surely she was kidding! She must be kidding! This was some kind of a game--a tug-of-war--and I was supposed to get Chedge away from her!

"Move, Sharon. I'll rescue Chedge!"

I slipped into the narrow space beside my mother and tried to reach behind.

Whack! Whack! Whack! She brought the stuffed toy down on my head once, twice, three times. I looked at her in surprise, then tried to grab the bear away.

"Go on! Get out of here, you two devils! I'll teach you to disobey!"

She chased us from the room, then slammed and locked the door.

Five, ten, fifteen minutes we waited outside that door, turning the knob, knocking softly, begging for forgiveness.

We heard the door of the incinerator creak open, and Mother empty a wastebasket into it, knocking it against the burner to remove every bit of trash.

Twice more the incinerator creaked open. Then, for a long time, there was silence.

Finally, Mother stepped out.

"Where's Chedge?" Sharon's voice shook with despair.

"Never mind where Chedge is. You don't deserve to know."

"Yes we do. We didn't do anything wrong," she said. "Where is he?"

Mother thrust a wastebasket at each of us.

"Here. Go put these away. Go on, now, do as I say, or there won't be any Easter Baskets! Go on, now!"

We ran upstairs. Then we ran back down.

"Can we have Chedge now? Where is he?" Mother was busy hanging clothes and did not look at me.

"He's in a safe place. I put him away."

We ran to the red-walled furnace room to look. Together we lifted our father's heavy tool box, peered behind jars of nails and screws, went into the darkness behind the furnace to see if Mother had thrown the bear back there. While I stood lookout, Sharon even stretched on tiptoe and reached back to feel behind the row of Dad's books that we were forbidden to read.

Then Sharon and I stopped and looked at each other. Where could Chedge be? She glanced up at the ceiling.

"Paula," she whispered, "go get a chair from the laundry room. I think she put him up there, in the ceiling, in those rafters!"

I dragged one of the old black metal chairs to where Sharon was standing, and she clambered up.

"Is he there? Do you see him?" I tilted my head back to watch Sharon as she stood on tiptoe to look, then saw her bravely sweep her arm into the dark spaces, unmindful of the spiders lurking there.

"No," she said finally, sighing and jumping down. "He's not here."

"Well, then, where else could he be?"

We looked at each other, and then, almost as with one mind, at the incinerator beside us.

"You open it."

"No, you. I reached up there, where there are spiders. Now it's your turn."

I nodded, and, taking a deep breath, I swung back the heavy door. Together, we looked inside. There was no sign of the waste paper, no sign of Chedge. Together, we breathed a sigh of relief, then went to find Mother.

"Won't you give us Chedge now?" I pleaded, handing her a clothespin for the wet sheet she was hanging.

"No. I told you no."

"But we want him," I pleaded. "When can we have Chedge? You said you'd give him back if we were good."

Mother turned and looked at each of us.

"That's right," she said. "When you can learn to be good."

Chapter 3

Basement

It was about 4:30 p.m., suppertime during those winters growing up in Detroit. By that time the light coming in the side door would be fading into night. It was freezing cold outside, and the snow had accumulated and melted since Thanksgiving until now, in January, mounds of it, dirtied by the frost-blackened leaves and pebbles, lined the driveway and lay like ash about the stoop.

"Paula! Come here! I need you!"

My mother's voice rose over the drone of the Mix Master that was buzzing on the black and white metal table as she made batter for the waffles.

"What, Mommy? Can I taste the batter? Can I have a piece of bacon?"

"No--it's too close to supper. Keep your fingers out of that--they're dirty! Go down to the fruit cellar and see if there's any maple syrup down there. He'll be so damned mad if he has to go out again, I hope there's some down there. Look for it on one of the middle shelves, and be careful not to drop it. That's all I'd need is to have to clean up another mess after working in this house all day today."

"Why can't Sharon go? I don't want to go down there "

"Sharon's lying down. I'm asking you to go."

"Why can't she go with me? "

"She's lying down, I told you. You know that she's not well and can't do much. You should try to be more thoughtful. Be grateful you don't have her problem. Now stop arguing with me and go. Oh, and remember, you only put on the middle light. We don't need all six lights on down there. It's a waste of electricity and money."

I nodded and stepped down onto the landing. The dim bulb did not light all the steps; the last two were in darkness. There was no light until you turned the corner and put them on in the laundry room. I stood there staring down into the blackness, my teeth busy on a thumb nail, then turned in terror and tripped up the landing stairs into the bright, warm kitchen.

" Stumble bum! What is the matter with you?"

I looked up at my mother through my tears. Her freshly ironed slacks, her pale beige sweater, the black eyes and hair that made soft waves about her thin face were a blur. But I could tell that my mother stood, as she often did, with her hands on her hips, and that she was holding one of the thick wooden spoons with which she sometimes hit me.

"Where is he?"

I was beginning to cry harder.

"Where is who--your father? I don't know. Maybe he's in the living room reading the Free Press."

I ran to check.

"No, he's not there."

"Well--then I don't know where he is. Just do as you're told and go down there and get that syrup. I'll be up here working. Just remember that, if you get scared."

Hanging on to the bannister with both hands, I put my red leather Indian slippers with the white fur and beads carefully down on the first step. I hated those stairs. They were painted a flat, dark grey. They were of wood and had no backs, so that my feet sometimes slipped through them when I ran up in fright, and I would gouge and bruise my shins.

I went down slowly at first, then faster. Jumping off the last two steps, I hugged the wall, reaching around into the darkness, trying to count the switches so I could find the one in the middle that I was allowed to turn on.

In my haste, my panic, I swept my hand across the switch. The light flickered momentarily as I turned to look into the room; then it went out. But it was on long enough for me to see a figure, a dark figure crouched two feet away by the stove, fingers curled into claws hiding a face with a snarling grin.

I started to scream. Suddenly, out of the darkness, out of the pitch blackness came a low, deep roar. I thought of the growler in my teddy bear; was my teddy bear down here? Then something grabbed my arm and pulled me into the darkness. I screamed and reached out, sweeping at the light switches, missing them in my terror.

"Hey, it's me, it's me. "

My father was hugging me tightly and laughing.

"You shouldn't be afraid. Why are you afraid? Why did you scream? See, it's only me. When I'm with you there's nothing down here to be frightened of."

I held tight to my father's neck, smelling the remnants of his day, the cold, fresh air, the Old Spice that he bought at the grocery, his oily blond hair and the putty and grease he used after sanding copper fittings at the construction site.

He had not turned on a light, but it did not matter. I was calm now, his pats were calming me, first on my back and then lower, little pats on my butt, and his hand running up and down between my legs, the corduroy beginning to make the familiar whish-whish sound I liked to hear when I walked, and his kisses, on my cheeks, my eyes, my mouth, until I hesitantly pushed away when his tongue touched mine, afraid that he would think I did not love him, needing to turn on the light but afraid to do so.

"Dad? Dad! What are you doing down there with her so long?"

My mother's voice, hollow, echoing slightly as it came down the stairs from the landing where she stood peering into the darkness, made my father relinquish his hold. I squirmed away and felt for the correct switch. He still crouched by the stove in his dark green work uniform and muddy leather boots, his soft yellow hair slightly mussed.

"Tell your mother it's o.k. Tell her you're looking for the syrup."

His whisper made me feel like a confederate, as if we were playing a secret prank upon my mother.

I giggled and called up the stairs, "It's o.k., Mommy. Daddy's down here with me."

"Yeah? I'll bet he is. He better leave you alone. If someone finds out about him, they'll lock him up. Dad, do you hear me? You better watch out, or she's going to end up in Northville in some kind of padded cell, and you'll be there right along with her!"

My father's laugh felt warm on my ear.

"Don't listen to her. She's mad because she didn't get to go downtown shopping."

I nodded my understanding.

"Will you stay down here with me while I look in the fruit cellar for some syrup?"

"Well, sure I will. In fact, we can look together!"

He took my small hand in his big one and helped me pull open the heavy, creaking, cobwebbed cellar door.

"Here's that old maple syrup, right here on the shelf."

He handed down a jug of Log Cabin from the top row, above his head. "Now, go on and take this up to your mother before she yells at you again. You're in enough trouble already."

Chapter 4

The Sparrow

I sat in the grey chair, trying to push my stuffed bear's paw through a sleeve too small for his furry arm. Pushing and pulling at it, I finally put the flannel nightie on him, tugged it around, straightened the material, and then held him up for inspection.

I giggled. "Look, Mother, Mr. Mole looks like a sausage!"

Mother glanced over her shoulder. "Uh-huh," she said absentmindedly. "You're feeling better, aren't you, honey?"

"Yep. Me and Mr. Mole are getting better!"

"Well, what a relief. My! So sick with all those chicken pox--chicken pox everywhere--on your eyelids, in your ears, your mouth, between your toes! And how many did we count on Sharon? Seven, was it? She brings them home and hardly gets sick and you nearly die from them. Some sister you have, eh my little Paula? Well, I'm glad it's over. It will be good to get some peace and sleep for once instead of taking care of sick kids all night long."

I said nothing. I sat watching my mother in the pearl-grey light of the morning as she reached to brush the cobwebs from the window corners and dusted the china swans and the porcelain shoes on the pink marble windowsills.

All of a sudden a shadow fell across the window and something hit it once, twice, three times.

Mother squealed. "Get away! Get away!" she said, her voice quivering as she waved her dust cloth at the window.

"What is it, Mother? Is a bat trying to get in the house?"

"No. It's a bird. A sparrow. It's trying to get in! "

Mother picked up the yellow dustmop and started shaking it at the window.

"But it can't get in. The window's closed!"

"Oh, if it's supposed to, it will find a way, down the chimney or something. Get away! Get away!"

The sparrow continued to fly at the window, pecking the newly washed panes with its beak.

"If it finds a way in--" Mother continued to flap furiously at the window with her dust cloth-- "it means one of us is going to die. My mother--Grandma--always said so."

"She did?" Mr. Mole fell to the floor as I jumped up and ran to my mother's side.

"Here! Leave me alone! I know, we'll close all the drapes!"

She ran from one window to the next until the three floor-length drapes were closed. Then she fell into a chair.

I gathered Mr. Mole up and stood next to her.

"Mother, who's going to die? Am I going to die?"

"No, you're better now, and so is Sharon. And your father never gets sick. He's too mean."

"You're not going to die, are you Mother?" I could feel the warm tears rising. "Please don't die and leave me."

"No? And why shouldn't I? I'm tired unto death right now, let me tell you, after staying up all week with a sick kid!"

"I'm sorry. I won't get sick again! If I do, I'll take care of myself! Please don't die and leave me."

I pushed my face into Mr. Mole's soft warm mohair to smother a sob.

"Don't cry. Why are you crying? Save your tears for when you'll really need them, Paula."

Mother stood up and moved to the picture window where she groped for the drapery cord.

"No, Mother! Please don't open the drapes."

"Are you crazy? We can't leave them shut in broad daylight. What would the neighbors think?"

"I don't care about them," I sobbed. "Don't let the sparrow come in!"

Mother looked at me and sighed. As she reached for the drapery cord, she began singing the hymn she always sang at times like this:

"On a hill far away stood an old rugged cross, the emblem of suff'ring and shame; and I love that old cross where the dearest and best, for a world of lost sinners was slain..."

She pulled the front drapes open and moved to one of the narrow side windows.

"No, Mother, no! Not those drapes, please don't open them! Please stop singing that song. I don't want you to die!"

Mother looked at me and laughed.

"You're feeling a lot better, aren't you? Just listen to you squeal! Now leave me alone!"

She pulled the second cord, hard, and the drapes swayed against the wall as they flew open.

"There! See? No birds. Now stop your crying."

"But the bird was here, at this window!"

I ran and stood between my mother and the wall.

"Let me in there, Paula. Get out of the way, you nut!"

I stood there stubbornly, hugging my teddy bear.

"So I'll cherish the old rugged cross, 'til my trophies at last I lay down..."

"No, Mother, please stop singing."

"That's a hymn, you little heathen. First you nearly tire me to death with your chicken pox, and now you're trying to keep me from God. Now, move!"

Mother reached out and pulled my hair sharply. I held up Mr. Mole to ward her off, and shrank away from the window. She reached behind the last drape, and with a quick, swift tug, it too, spread wide. The sparrow was gone. I felt an instant relief.

Mother turned and picked up her dust rag.

"I will cling to that old rugged cross, and exchange it someday for a crown."

Chapter 5

The Good
Humor Man

"Daddy, what time is it, please?"

I pressed my forehead against the screen door in my parents' room that led to the backyard where my dad knelt, spreading peat moss among the roses.

"I don't know, Paula. My watch is in the house. Go look at the clock."

"I just did, but I'm not sure. I'm just learning how to tell time."

Dad did not look up. He continued to dip his broad hands in the black peat and spread it deftly around the flowers.

"Could you come in and see, Daddy, please? I'd ask Sharon, but she's in the bathroom, and I want to know now."

"Why? Are you going somewhere?"

"No, Daddy!" I giggled. "I want to see if it's one o'clock yet, because that's when Art comes everyday."

"Who?"

"You know, the ice cream man in the white truck. Can we have ice cream, Daddy? It's so hot today."

He did not answer. He was examining the branches of a pink rose, running his fingers along them and then wiping his hands on his pants.

"What are you doing, Daddy?"

"Oh, these bushes have little green bugs called aphids, and this is a way to kill them before they eat the plants. Come outside and I'll show you."

"But I just have my panties on. I have to stay in the house."

Just then, Sharon joined me at the back door. We cupped our eyes and peered at our father through the dark screen.

"Dad, it's almost one o'clock when the ice cream man comes. Can Paula and I have money for a Good Humor bar?"

"How much is it?"

"Ten cents."

"Ten cents; you mean a nickle apiece?"

"No, Daddy, ten cents each."

"Ten cents each! How many ice creams do you get for a dime?"

"Just one. We could each get two halves, but Mother won't let us eat popsicles. She says they cause sore throats."

Suddenly we heard the bell on Art's truck jingle as he wended his way down Mansfield.

"Please, Daddy? Can we have ice cream?"

"Hurry, Daddy!" Sharon pleaded. "He's in the next block and we have to go put on our shirts and shorts before he comes!"

"Why do you have to do that?"

Dad sat back on his heels and squinted in at us.

"Because we can't go get ice cream in our underpants."

The jingle of the bell drew nearer.

"Please, Daddy!"

"Do you like popsicles?"

Sharon and I nodded.

"We had them at Grandma's every day when we stayed with her last week, and we didn't get a sore throat once. Mother always makes us get orange creamsicles. She says the vanilla ice cream must be good for us, because that's what they have in the hospital. We eat it, but we don't really like it."

Suddenly I squealed. The ice cream truck was getting closer.

"Would you girls like popsicles this time?"

I glanced up at my sister. Sharon looked worried.

"But we'll get in trouble with Mother if we have popsicles, won't we?"

"We won't tell her," he said. "Then she can't get mad. But you won't be able to get dressed. You'll have to go out to the street in your panties."

The bell on the ice cream truck jangled wildly. Art was waiting at the curb.

Sharon hesitated.

"I guess we don't want any ice cream today."

Our father opened his palm. The silver shone in the summer sun.

"Popsicles? Our secret treat?"

He shook the coins like dice.

Suddenly we each grabbed a dime, hugged our dad, then ran through the house toward the street.

Chapter 6

Boys' Names

"If you and your sister ever get married, be sure that you have sons," my mother would sometimes caution me. "Men don't feel like men unless they have sons."

"Daddy has us. He seems to be happy."

"With Sharon, maybe. She was the first born. The first one is always special, no matter what it is. But you. You were supposed to be a boy."

"Daddy likes me, even if I'm not."

"Yeah? Well, he'd like you better if you were a boy. You were going to be Paul, after him and Grandpa Miner, but when he saw what you were he just shrugged and said to name you Paula.

"And that was that. No more kids. I tried and tried, but all I could have was two girls. Just girls. I often think..."

Mother's voice trailed off as she paused in her work.

"Think what, Mother?" I looked up at her, eager for what was to come.

"Oh, nothing. Never mind. Here. Fold these clothes for me."

I tried again. "Think what, Mommy?"

"Oh," she sighed heavily. "Just that things would be different if the boy had lived. You know, he was really the first baby, a little boy. We had the name all picked out. Mark. Little Mark. Marky."

"How did he die? Is he in Heaven with Jesus?"

"I had a miscarriage at five months and lost him. He'd be, let's see, you're seven and Sharon's almost ten. Gee, he'd be a teenager now. Wouldn't that have been wonderful, to have had a son. But instead we got Sharon, and then you came along. Another girl."

"Maybe you can have a baby boy now. Can I have a baby brother?"

"I guess it just wasn't meant to be. No, no more kids. Even two is too many."

Chapter 7

The Monkey and the Weasel

"All around the cobbler's bench, the monkey chased the weasel! The monkey stopped to pull up his socks. Pop! Goes the weasel!"

As the arm on the little record player scratched to the end of the record and moved back and forth crazily out of track, I paused to reset it.

"Hurry, Paula, hurry! Daddy's going to catch you!"

Mother stood bathed in the light by the kitchen sink, laughing over her shoulder at the antics in the dark dining room.

"Oh, oh! I better watch out!"

I dropped the arm on the bright red plastic record. The voice wavered, then began again as I galloped around the big mahogany table. I looked over my shoulder, panting. Daddy was coming, his big hands and short, broad fingers splayed on the carpeting as he crawled rapidly behind me, growling.

"Here I come, little weasel. The monkey's coming to get you!"

Round and round the table we went, faster and faster. I was breathing hard, and the slippery feet in my worn red sleepers slid on the carpeting. I fell on one knee.

Suddenly I felt Daddy's thumb, once, twice.

I scrambled to my feet.

"Stop that! Mother, tell him to stop goosing me. I don't like that."

"Paul," Mother called from the kitchen, "what did I tell you about that? If you don't leave her alone, one day the little men in the white coats with the butterfly nets are going to catch you and Paula and haul you both away to Northville."

A metal pot my mother was rinsing bumped the porcelain sink.

"It's only a game," Daddy said near me in the dark room.

"Come on, let's play."

"Uh-uh. I'm pooped. I need to sit down."

"Here. Sit here, on my lap."

Daddy leaned against the wall and reached for me but he missed. His hand caught the back of my sleepers. The trap door fell down.

"Oh, what's this? A moon! The weasel's moon! Isn't it cute?"

He cupped my buttocks in his hands.

"No, Daddy. Don't!"

I squirmed away as he grabbed for my leg, and ran toward the light in the kitchen.

"Why is your trapdoor down?"

I pulled the material around, trying to snap it.

"I can't get it snapped. Will you help me, Mother?"

"No. Here you are, almost eight years old and you still can't take care of yourself. Maybe if you'd stop biting your nails down to the quick, your fingers would work better. As it is, you're nothing but a bumblefingers. Anyway, my hands are all wet. I only have a few more dishes to wash, and then I can go sit down and rest. I don't want to stop now. Go ask your father. He'll help you."

Daddy crawled to the kitchen door and growled.

I screamed and ran to the bathroom, slamming the door.

"Stop slamming that door!" Mother yelled after me. "What's gotten into her anyway? Do you know, Paul? Here you were, playing so nice with her, and she's acting like a nut again. I just don't know about that one. She sure isn't anything like Sharon!"

I leaned against the door, trying desperately to close the snaps, afraid that Daddy would come in. I couldn't get them to snap. I pressed my ear to the door and listened. Daddy was helping Mother dry the dishes.

I quietly opened the bathroom door, held the seat of my sleepers closed with one hand, and tiptoed down the hallway to my room. I rummaged in my middle dresser drawer, pulled out underpants and pajamas, and quickly changed clothes. Then I took the red sleepers and hid them in the narrow space between the dresser and the wall.

I took my fuzzy pink robe from the closet, wrapped it tightly around me, and made a double knot in the tie around my waist. Then I cautiously opened the bedroom door. I could hear my parents talking softly in the kitchen, their voices a comforting murmur. I walked quickly down the hall, crossed the kitchen and stood close to my mother on the other side from my father.

Mother's head was down near the sink as she scrubbed the under side of the faucet with cleanser, so she did not look at me.

"Did you finally snap those sleepers, Paula?"

"No," I mumbled.

"What? Speak up. I can't hear you."

"She said 'no'." My father answered for me. "She didn't snap the sleepers. Instead of asking for help, she changed into her pajamas."

Mother straightened and looked down at me.

"Why are you all bundled up like that? Where are your sleepers?"

I looked at the floor and shrugged.

"Come on, tell me! What did you do with those sleepers?"

"They're in the bedroom."

"Here you put on clean sleepers first and then you go back and dirty even more clothes putting on clean pajamas!" Mother cleared her throat angrily. "You'll be the death of me, Paula, making all that extra wash for me to do. Why couldn't you just come in here and let me or Daddy help you? Why is it always so hard to ask us for help when you need it?"

Again, I made no reply.

"Well, I want those clean pajamas off and the sleepers back on. Go on, right now. Go."

"Will you help me snap them, Mother?" I looked up at her through tear-filled eyes.

"No. Can't you see I'm still not through in this damned kitchen? I'm like a prisoner in here. Your dad will help you.

"Paul, go on, go dress her. And then put her to bed when you're finished."

Chapter 8

Suicide

The first time I tried to kill myself, I was only eight years old.

I stood in the dark hallway just outside the partially closed door of the bedroom I shared with my older sister. As I examined my fingers, looking for a new shred of flesh or nail to tear into, I listened to my mother talk to my sister.

"Poor little Sharon! Why did God ever have to punish you like this, making you so sickly all the time? My, my. I just don't get it. Something so small and happy and innocent and kind hearted. If it had been your sister, always fighting with you, always so mean to you, then I'd understand. But you!"

As I stood in the dark, listening, my eyes filled, and a sob caught in my throat.

"Who's there? Dad? Is that you? Can you see, Sharon? I'll bet he's out there peeking through the crack of the door at us again!"

Sharon leaned forward in her bed to look.

"No, it's only Paula."

"Paula? Come here, honey."

I slowly entered, my head down.

"Are you crying?"

I shrugged.

"Why are you crying? Are you still mad that you had to do the dinner dishes? Don't you understand your sister is sick again and has to rest?" Mother let out a sigh of exasperation.

"When will you get it through your thick head how lucky you are to have good health? You're just like your father, so stubborn!"

I started to cry, hard.

"Now, stop your crying! Stop it, or I'll give you something to cry about! Here, take this Kleenex and blow your nose."

Mother tossed a yellow tissue to me. I scooped it up as it reached the floor.

"That's better. Now, do you want to hear a story? Sharon asked me to read to her from 'Mrs. Piggle Wiggle.'"

"Can't you read from my new Uncle Wiggly book instead?"

"No, she asked for 'Mrs. Piggle Wiggle', didn't you honey? Besides, that Uncle Wiggly is for you to read by yourself. Miss Craciola said if you don't start reading by yourself, even if it's only your baby books, you'll be a flunky all the way through school and end up like that girl up the street there, pregnant at 16."

I stood at the foot of my sister's bed, saying nothing, watching.

Mother had tucked the warm blankets around Sharon and turned the green hobnail bedspread back neatly, so that the bed made me think of a picture in a magazine. Sharon sat forward for a moment to pull one of the pillows out from behind her for Mother to lean against, and together they leafed through 'Mrs. Piggle Wiggle,' laughing at the pictures and selecting a story. Finally, Mother looked up.

"Well," she said to me. "Are you going to listen or not?"

I shrugged.

"It's getting late, and I can't wait forever for you to make up your mind. Oh, did you empty the wastebaskets after you finished the dishes, like I told you?"

I shook my head. No.

"Why not? Did you forget?"

I shook my head. Yes.

"Stop biting your nails and answer me!"

"I'm sorry. I forgot."

"Then go do it right now, like I told you."

"Where's Dad?"

"Why?"

"I don't know, I was just wondering."

"Every time I ask you to do something for me, you want to know where he is. Why? Are you still afraid of bogymen? Grow up, Paula. There's nothing down there. Now, go."

I stood, looking at my mother as she leant back against one of the pillows my sister had plumped for her.

"What is it now?"

"Well. . . Where's Dad?"

"He's in bed. Asleep. Are you satisfied? Now go and do what I told you to do, and be quiet. Don't make a lot of racket when you get my wastebasket out."

"O.K. If I hurry, will you wait until I get back to read from 'Mrs. Piggle Wiggle'?"

"I don't know. We'll see. Just hurry up."

I grabbed the wastebasket in our room, carefully opened the door to my parents' room across the narrow hall, then waited, listening. I could hear my father's even breaths, huh...sss huh...sss. I crept in, grabbed the metal basket from its usual position behind the door, and was making a careful arc to bring it from the room when it suddenly caught a corner of the dresser. There was a clank of dull metal.

"Shhh! You'll wake him!"

"Hey! What are you doing? Who's making that noise?"

"It's o.k., Dad, go back to sleep. It's nothing. Paula needed something."

"Well, I have to get up early, you know..."

"Paula? Did you hear him? Quit making so much noise!" My mother's voice hissed down the hall.

I tiptoed into the bathroom, picked up that basket, and emptied it into one of the bedroom receptacles. Then I picked up the metal basket and our plastic one in my right hand, ran through the kitchen, took up the large red kitchen wastebasket in my left hand, turned the stairway light on with my elbow, hesitated on the top step, then hurried down.

In my haste I missed the second to the last step, lost my footing and went down, grazing my tailbone on the last riser. The metal basket clanged loudly, once, as it hit the cement floor. I cringed, waiting for my mother's angry voice to echo from my bedroom through the heating duct overhead, but there was nothing, nothing now but silence from the musty basement.

I rose slowly, new tears stinging my eyes. Not only had I botched the chore and hurt myself, but Mother would be angered by the delay, by my clumsiness, which she had surely heard.

I stood there for a minute looking into the darkness of the laundry room, took a deep breath, reached for the middle switch, gathered up the spilled trash, then limped through to the furnace room and the incinerator where we burned our refuse.

I dumped the waste into the incinerator. The blue flame of gas flared orange as I blew softly at it so that it would ignite and burn the trash. Then I looked around at the screwdrivers, drills, hammers and saws my father had hung everywhere on the red walls, in another quick and desperate search for Chedge.

I peered behind the jars of nails and screws on the shelves that lined one wall, then peeked into the dark place behind the furnace. I was certain I would find him. But I couldn't find him this time, either, so I gathered the empty wastebaskets, jumped up to catch the light cord next to the bulb, raced through the half dark laundry room, rounded the corner and scrambled upstairs.

It was quiet at the back of the house.

"Oh, good," I thought to myself, "She hasn't started reading yet."

The sound of quiet laughter floated from the bedroom.

"Done, Mother. What story will you read?"

"What do you mean, 'Will you read?' We're nearly finished. Sharon and I were just laughing at this picture."

Mother held up the book like the librarian in school during reading hour.

"What are they doing there? What's the story about?"

"Never mind. It would take longer to tell you than it would to read it again."

"Oh, will you?"

"Will I what?"

"Read it again. I've never heard that story. Please?"

"Are you crazy? It's nearly nine o'clock, and Sharon needs her rest, don't you, honey? And you do, too, Paula. Let me finish these two pages, comb Sharon's hair and yours, and then it will be time to go to sleep."

"But you promised you'd wait! You said if I hurried you'd wait to read the story!"

"I said no such thing. Besides, you took too damn long, making all that noise, waking your father up, then falling down the stairs. Did you get hurt?"

I nodded, rubbing my spine. I could not speak. Already new tears were catching in my throat.

"Well, it serves you right. Always in a hurry, Paula. That's why your legs usually look so bruised and ugly."

"But Mother, you told me to..."

"Never mind. Don't argue. Now, go bring my comb and brush from off my dresser. Sharon, if you can turn the pages I can finish the story and fix your hair at the same time."

I stopped my ears with my fingers and ran from the room. A moment later, I returned, but instead of handing the white nylon comb to my mother, I threw it at her. It hit her in the chest.

"You threw it at me! Did you see that? She threw that comb at me like a knife! You hate me, don't you, Paula? I bet you wish that comb were a knife so you could murder me. Look at that red mark, Sharon--like a knife wound in the chest!"

I ran from the room crying.

"No, no," I sobbed. "I'm sorry, Mother! I was throwing it to you! I thought you'd catch it! I'm sorry I hurt you!"

I ran into the bathroom, put on the light, and locked the door. My mother's angry shouts--"Murderer! Murderer!" rang in my ears.

I turned the water in the sink on hard to drown her out, then looked up into the mirror at my snot-covered, swollen red face. I hated myself, so stupid, so ugly, the tears and snots mingling with drool that fell from my lips.

I had tried to kill my mother! Never mind that it was with a comb, not a knife! Had I thrown it? I just meant to toss it, but Mother said I had thrown it, and she knew, didn't she? Hadn't she felt it? Hadn't it hurt? I had tried to kill her!

Thinking wildly what to do, I pulled opened the door to the medicine chest. There was mother's razor, the one we were forbidden to touch. There was the bottle of iodine, the one with the skull and cross bones. There was the new bottle of aspirin, the kind Mother took for her arthritis.

I grabbed the bottle and pulled out the cotton; five, ten pills spilled into my hand. I smashed them into my mouth, took huge gulps of water, then took another handful. At last, only three were left.

I had stopped crying. After I splashed water on my face and dried it hard on one of the dainty, embroidered fingertip towels, some of the redness disappeared.

I opened the door softly, quietly, and went back into the bedroom.

"What were you doing in there so long?"

I shrugged at my mother, my back to her as I climbed into bed.

"Huh? Answer me! What were you doing in there so long?"

My mother had turned to tuck the covers in around my sister. She bent down, tickled Sharon, then gave her a kiss goodnight.

"Well?"

Mother was over me now, pulling the covers up firmly under my chin.

"I was in the bathroom. I...I took your whole bottle of aspirin. I only saved you three."

"You took all that aspirin? What were you trying to do, kill yourself?"

For a moment our eyes locked. I nodded.

"Well, you'll never do it with aspirin. It's not strong enough."

Then she turned, clicked off the light and went out.

Chapter 9

Hospital Corners

"No, that's not right. Smoother. No wrinkles!"

Mother jerked the white cotton sheet off the twin bed mattress and threw it on the floor at my feet.

"Again! Do it again! And this time, do it right, or I'll spank you! Sharon's making her bed look perfect. Why can't you?"

I watched my sister slip the unfitted bottom sheet under the mattress at the foot of her bed, pull the corner of the fabric toward her, fold it envelope fashion, then tuck it in.

"There! How's that?" Sharon beamed up at Mother.

"Those are perfect hospital corners, Sharon. See how smooth that sheet is? Paula says she wants to be a nurse, but nurses have to know how to make beds right. Maybe Sharon will be the nurse, and Paula will carry the bedpans."

I fought back the tears. "But Sharon's bigger. She can reach across her bed to smooth her sheet. I'm too little. I still need help."

Mother was on her way out the bedroom door.

"Shut up, Paula--stop talking back. If you're old enough to be in Kindergarten, you're old enough to change your bed properly. And don't go to Sharon for help as soon as my back is turned. Remember, Paula, the Lord helps those who help themselves."

Chapter 10

Education

Mother and Dad put our Capart console television with the 12 inch screen just to the left of the big picture window in the living room. At night we closed the rose-colored drapes that exactly matched the walls and the cabbage roses in the carpeting. Sharon and I would argue briefly over whose turn it was to sit in the boxy chair by the television, and Mother and Dad would select the programs.

There may have been other choices, but the shows my family watched were situation comedies--*The Jackie Gleason Show*, *Amos N' Andy*, *The Life of Riley*. It was these shows, and my parents' comments that taught me about sexual attitudes and social behavior, about blacks and ethnic groups-- and about something more.

"Alice, Alice, one of these days, Alice! Pow! Right in the kisser!"

Ralph Kramden's words became a catch phrase of the 60s. Boys would accost girls on grade school playgrounds, make a fist and threaten to send the giggling little Alices to the moon. Sharon and I would repeat the game at home. When our aunts and uncles came to visit, they would laugh with Mother and Dad about the antics of *The Honeymooners*, each time playing out the scenario between Ralph and Alice.

"Geez," Dad said, "isn't that guy something, always threatening his wife like that? Oh, man."

"Well, Alice asks for it," Mother replied. "She's forever talking back to him. He ought to haul off and let her have it once, good. Then she wouldn't be so mouthy, such a witch. Aren't you glad you're not married to someone like her?"

Ralph Kramden frightened me. Alice Kramden fascinated me. He was loud and brash, as we were not. He was menacing. So was my mother. His threats were akin to hers; the fist he held in Alice's face was my mother's hand, sweeping back in anger, then, fueled by the power of her sudden rage, almost splitting my cheek, my mouth in two.

What fascinated me about Alice was how she would not be bullied. I can see her now in the dilapidated little tenement apartment, jaw set, hands on hips, yelling back at her husband. And there was the difference. Alice and Ralph shared common ground. But I was at the mercy of my mother. I was not allowed to express whatever anger I felt, to shout back or to strike back, for these were the earmarks of poor breeding and of the supreme breach of parental respect.

So I would stand there with my head bowed, another wash of angry tears spilling over me as my mother began her familiar rebuke.

"You big, stupid oaf! Don't you ever talk back to your mother ever again, or I'll knock your head off!" my mother often shouted in her rage. "Look at you! I can hardly reach you any more to punish you, you gargantuan! You're going to grow up to be an Amazon and then I'll have to wallop you extra hard. So remember that! Remember what's coming the next time you lip off!"

And so, with my head hanging, I would agree with every word my mother said about how bad I was, agree again and again with those hard words that inevitably followed those swift smacks because she, after all, was my mother. If she didn't know the truth about me, then who did? And every time this happened, it would trigger that sustaining, that comforting thought: I'm going to kill myself.

"Those stupid niggers!" Mother said repeatedly about Amos and Andy, whose antics reinforced the prevaling views among white Americans of blacks as lazy and ignorant. "Did you see what he just did?" Her head fell back as she laughed at a weekly television episode.

"And Ruby Begonia! Cheez!" Dad's shoulders shook with laughter at the dilemmas that she, Sapphire and the men inevitably found themselves in.

"Oh well," he'd say, shrugging, "just another big, fat stupid nigger."

"Yeah. They're all like that," Mother agreed. "Fat and lazy. And that King Fish. Isn't he a crook? And those other stupid niggers fall for it every time! They should ship them all back to Africa where they belong."

I liked to watch the program to hear my parents laugh. But, perhaps because I was so often the object of my parents' derision, I empathized with the people they laughed at. I hated King Fish, not because he was black, but because he took advantage of such nice, unsuspecting people. And although Ruby Begonia was fat--a favorite indictment of my svelte mother--to me she seemed good natured and kind, rather than dumb. I liked her, I liked all the people on the show except for the shysters, the sharps who each week conned and swindled those they saw as inferior.

Perhaps that is why I asked for--and received--a black baby doll for Christmas when I was four or five, a baby doll I dressed, diapered, fed, talked and sang to and took everywhere with me--to the living room, to the kitchen, to the basement--but never into the backyard or for a ride around the block in the doll buggy because it wasn't allowed. When I asked my dad why I couldn't take my doll to church, he laughed and replied, "You wouldn't want to do that now, would you?"

I stopped playing with my black baby altogether the Christmas I got a brand new doll. She wore a pink pique dress and a pink cotton bonnet with a firmly starched brim. She could go with me everywhere. She was white.

Television also nurtured my parents' sense of ethnic superiority. Consider the weekly predicaments of that well-intentioned, rather inept middle class white male on *The Life of Riley*. Because of his large nose and work uniforms, I kept thinking that Riley was my father, that somehow Dad could be sitting on the couch with Mother, pointing and laughing at the ignorance of this man, and, at the very same moment, be living in another house with another dark-haired wife named Peg. It took my parents a long time to convince me that I was really seeing two different men, because one was a "stupid Mick," and the other was my father.

And what were my parents? They were the children of Slav and Russian immigrants who came over to America on the boat, knowing no English and with only the vaguest sense of where it was they were going and what they were about. I guess that made my grandparents DPs--displaced persons--another common taunt--but one that was never applied to members of my own family, or to me. But everyone else, it seemed, was fair game.

They would make fun of people--my great uncle Pete who was bent nearly in two by the arthritis in his spine, the family of 14 to whom we gave hand-me-downs, the missionaries who came to speak at Alpha Baptist Church, the deaf man who sold the Free Press at Livernois and McNichols in Detroit.

Away from home, writing and music became the outlets for my pent-up rage. To their credit, my parents recognized early that I had musical talent, and financed years of lessons in piano, violin and viola-- the very instruments they had only dreamed of learning as Depression-era children. Music teachers discovered I have perfect pitch and natural singing ability. At Detroit's Cooley High School and Wayne State University, I spent my time cleansing my soul by participating in small, audition-only vocal ensembles, by singing radio and television commercials, and by writing for the student newspapers.

I needed those emotional outlets to protect me from what went on at home. If I sang, my parents would cover their ears and cringe, or howl like injured dogs. Or, if we had company, I would be invited to play the piano, then I would be begged, and then, ordered. Everyone would be quiet, waiting, watching. Someone, my mother or father, would coax me.

"Play something short, Paula. You play so well. Go ahead, honey, we want to hear you."

Thus reassured, I would begin playing some well-practiced favorite. But when I made a mistake, which I invariably did, my parents would begin.

"Ouch! Mozart must be turning over in his grave!"

"Did you hear that, Dad? That was a really big goof."

More mistakes.

"Hey, bumble fingers!" It was a favorite nickname of my father's. "You're supposed to be playing with your fingers, not your fists."

And so it would go, until, blinded by tears of rage, embarrassment, and trust denied, I would jump up and run out of the room crying, too humiliated to face my relatives at the dinner table, believing that my parents were right, for just look at all the mistakes I had made!

I learned a great deal from my parents during those growing up years in Detroit: how to submit to abuse, how to hate blacks, Irishmen and others, how to belittle the disabled, how to question my native talents. But mostly what I learned was how not to be.

Chapter 11

Anger Turned Inward

Depression is anger turned inward. The greater the anger, and the longer you have felt this anger, the greater the depression will be. Many of us have been taught that the expression of anger is wrong; that it is not gentlemanly or ladylike to get mad, or that it is unChristian. So we learn to stuff our rages, our negatives, our hostilities deep within us. When we raise up our eyes, they are troubled, they are clouded, they see fire and are alight with it.

Anger is a legitimate emotion; all of God's creatures express anger. Consider the blue jay, railing at the house cat from a tree. Consider the German shepherd that snarls and bites at anyone who carries a shovel or a rake because it was beaten with the tools as a pup.

These are images from nature; these creatures are things of beauty, just as each of us is a splendid and beautiful expression born out of the love the Creator has for every thing in the universe, for God does not make junk.

And yet our anger interferes with our beauty, stops us from seeing correctly, stops us from being and becoming. We must unclench our fists, we must heave the deepest sighs we have ever breathed--so deep that they shake the earth--we must scream the loudest screams, cry the greatest cries of anguish that the universe has ever heard in order to shake this anger from us. We must cry, cry today, cry tomorrow, cry for two, for three years in order to let the anger flow out from us so that peace can enter in.

It was my therapist in Nashville, Tennessee, who said to me three years ago, "Do you know how angry you look?" I turned from her and glanced in a mirror--in those days I was barely able to raise my eyes to look myself in the face.

"No," I told her, "I don't know. I can't see it. This is simply me that I see. This is how I've always looked."

And I felt angry at her for asking me that question, for telling me I looked angry. I didn't seek her out to get help for anger; I went to her because I was so severely depressed that I could no longer function, but would sit long hours on the couch in my apartment with but one thought on my mind--to kill myself.

"No," I said, sorrowfully, quietly, for I had already stored the rage I felt toward this question and toward her somewhere deep within me. "No, I don't look angry."

It was then that the tears started flowing from the depths of my heart, my being, my soul. They haven't stopped, and I cry now, even as I write. For more than three years I couldn't look into the eyes of anyone, so great was the despair within me. Nor could I unclench my fists or unfurrow my brow. I wanted to desperately, but I didn't know how.

I brought those tears, that rage with me to Bowling Green, Kentucky. It was the only way I knew how to be. Nobody had ever taught me to express my anger in a positive way. Rather, I had been taught that what I felt or thought was unimportant. Nobody really wanted to hear about my problems, so nobody did. With no place else to go, my negative feelings went deep inside, and began to eat me up.

As a child, an adolescent, a teenager sometimes the angry feelings would well up in me and spill out in words, and then my mother would brand me a rebel, an incorrigible, a delinquent, and she would slap me as hard as possible across the face.

"There," her actions said, "keep your anger to yourself."

Little by little during those growing up years, as my anger, my blame turned inward, I began to see myself as despicable, worthless, an ever greater object of my own hatred. Why should one such as I want to live? My focus became suicide, my life's purpose, to die.

How was I to know, as an adult, that not everybody in the world would see and behave toward me as my parents did? It has taken me years to discover this, bit by bit, as one peels away the layers of an onion.

But as I began to observe--and to admit-- that people actually found me interesting, intelligent, kind, spiritual, and something of a comedian, it felt as if some rare and amazing tomb of treasures was opening to me-- so rarefied, in fact, that for a long time I believed it to be a mirage; I tested and retested the loving guardians of this treasure house to see if they weren't tricksters or ghosts.

Chapter 12

Tiny Tears

"Paula, what do you want for Christmas? Sharon has already made out her list, and she's got a million things on it, as usual. Now, I know you aren't greedy and selfish like she is, but there must be something you want. Is there? Something special, I mean."

I hesitated. Should I tell her about the one thing I wanted more than anything else? What if she laughed? She would laugh! But if I didn't tell her, I wouldn't get that one thing that I longed for.

"There is something I really want, but it's probably too expensive. But I really want it more than anything in the whole world!"

I had my mother's attention. "Well, what is it?"

I looked down at my shoes. "You'll think it's dumb."

"No, I won't, honey, tell me. If you don't tell me, how will I know what to get for you?"

"Aw, all right." I took a deep breath, gripped my hands tightly behind my back, and blurted out my dream gift. "I want a Tiny Tears doll for Christmas."

"A Tiny Tears doll, for an Amazon like you? When are you going to grow up, Paula? You're almost twelve years old and still playing with dolls! Sometimes I really worry about you."

"But Mother, you asked me what I wanted, and that's it. That's all I want. I love dolls, and you said yourself that girls who love to play with dolls always make the best mothers. So I'll be a good mother when I grow up!"

"When are you going to get interested in jewelry and clothes, like your sister? I bet none of your girlfriends plays with dolls. And if the boys in your room knew, they'd laugh at you."

"But they won't know, because nobody will tell them. I'd just play with her in my room, and not even my girlfriends will know." I paused. "Please, Mother. That's all I want. I saw one the other day when I was waiting to meet you after work."

"You were in the Toy Department? Who said you could go to the Toy Department by yourself? Some big man is going to haul you into the stock room and strangle you and then, good-bye! You know you're supposed to come down the elevator and wait right by the refrigerators for me."

"Well, Dad took me to meet you one day last week, so I just went over to look at the dolls for a minute, and then I came right back. That's when I saw Tiny Tears. She's in a big box and she has on a little pink and white playsuit with her name embroidered in red and she has white booties and a baby bottle and a blue and pink rattle and a little blue and pink and white toy chest that says 'Tiny Tears' on it. Oh, and her arms were up, and it was just like she was asking to be hugged. And, and that's all I want." I held back the tears. "Please, Mother? And don't tell Dad that I was in the Toy Department instead of by the refrigerators, or he'll be really mad, okay?"

"Well, we'll see. He trusts you to go right to the door where I come out of work, and when you do somthing bad like not going there right away, you're being disobedient. I don't know. You probably should be punished. I'll have to think about it."

"Please don't tell. I won't go look at the toys again unless you're with me. I promise! But don't tell him!"

"Ha! When do we ever have a chance to do anything after work but rush right out to the car so he can get home and work on his stupid yard? That'll be the day when we can take five damn minutes to look at the toys, or anything else for that matter! And then the store closes 10 minutes after they let us out. Just like a damned prison! Prison at home, prison at work. Always the same damned thing!"

Christmas that year was like every Christmas I could remember: terrible, and perfect. For several years we'd had an artificial tree, but that year, after watching all the wonderful old sentimental movies like *Holiday Inn*, and *It's a Wonderful Life*, Sharon and I decided we had to have a live tree.

It always took forever to ask our father something; mother seemed less likely to rise to instant anger, to say "no" without first considering the request. Sometimes we got what we wanted-- ice cream or to go to the movies or to a friend's house. If she finally said "no" and we asked why, she would usually say, "Just because, that's all." Or, "Never mind. Don't ask so many questions. No means no. You don't need any explanations." Her other response to our timid requests was, "I don't know. Go ask your father, and quit bothering me already."

Asking Dad was much worse, and it usually took us a long time to get up our nerve to do it. We'd linger outside the room where he sat, reading a book or the paper, whispering, sometimes giggling in our fear.

"You go first."

"No, you."

"No. I went first and asked the last time. It's your turn." If a fight didn't erupt then and there between us, and if our arguments didn't disturb Dad to the point that we'd get yelled at before we made our request, one of us would push the other into the room and stammer out the question.

"Dad, will you drive us to a lot and help us pick out a live tree?"

"You've already got a tree. If you want to put one up this year, use the fake one."

"Please, Dad? Couldn't we have a real tree just once? It would make the house smell so good!"

"No. I told you we already have a tree. That's good enough. If you don't like that one, then do without."

We left the room with our heads and hearts downtrodden, went to our room, and muttered acrimoniously about Scrooge.

As luck would have it, that year someone put up a Christmas tree lot about a block and a half away on Six Mile Road. We hatched a plan: we'd do more work around the house to earn extra money, pool it, and buy our own live tree. But how to get it home?

"We can carry it!"

"But it'll be too heavy. Our arms will get tired."

"We can set it down and rest."

"We could pull it in the wagon!"

"But Dad put that in the attic of the garage. If we ask for it, he'll want to know why we want it, and if we tell him, he won't take it down."

We went to bed that night without a workable solution. We'd sleep on it.

In the morning, our answer was just outside the window. It had snowed. Now we could pull the tree on our sled.

"Just like in the old movies!"

"Yeah!"

We counted our money, waited for Mother and Dad to leave for work, and then set out. We paid a fortune for our tree--seven dollars--but it was worth it. It smelled so good we nearly hugged it. This would be the best Christmas ever!

Sharon and I worked all morning trying to get the tree in the stand. Finally we screwed it in crooked, reasoning that once our father saw how beautiful the tree looked and how good it smelled, he'd fix it for us.

We dressed it that afternoon. We had old, beautiful lights and ornaments, most of them from Germany, many dating back to World War I, mother would tell us--strings of lights with lanterns and parrots, fragile balls painted with stripes and stars, silver birds with feather tails, sparkling peaches, plums and grapes, and heavy foil tinsel which had to be carefully separated because we used it year after year. I placed the old cottony skirt around the tree stand, pinching it in places to hide the holes, while Sharon put the angel with the oil cloth skirt on the top branch. We stood back to admire our handiwork and gave each other a hug. It was beautiful, especially with the snow outside; it was just like *Christmas in Connecticut.*

We made a fire in the fireplace and, when Mother and Dad drove up, we lit the tree. We watched as Mother pointed and smiled. We watched Dad shrug his shoulders and shake his head. I could imagine him saying, "Ehh."

"That tree's crooked," Mother called as she entered the house.

"But don't you think it's beautiful? Don't you love the way it smells?"

"Your Dad's really mad because you went against his wishes. Just look at these boxes and papers! Clean up this mess before he comes in here. Paula, did you forget to start the dinner? Why didn't you kids decorate the mantle?"

Somehow the tree wasn't so much fun any more. We gathered up the ornament bags and boxes, vaccumed up the needles and tinsel, and hurried to get dinner going. Nothing more was said of the tree. By morning it stood straighter in its stand.

"Your dad really fumed at you kids last night, boy," Mother told us over cups of Ovaltine. "It took him about an hour to fix that stupid tree. Next time, do as you're told. Leave well enough alone."

Mother had wonderful taste and enjoyed buying us fine things. Sharon and I always got new outfits in addition to our Christmas dresses, and this year Mother chose soft wool skirts with matching, fur-blend cardigans for each of us. Sharon's was pale yellow, and mine, pale blue.

"Now, be very careful when you wear those things, because the skirts have to be dry cleaned," she cautioned as we pulled the outfits from the boxes. "Maybe I'll only let you wear those for good. I haven't decided yet."

There was a gold Florentine bracelet for Sharon, and a smooth silver bracelet with a chain guard for me, and a beautiful silver ring with a black pearl.

"Oh, thank you!" I gasped as I tried them on. "These are beautiful! How did you know I like silver?"

"Silver is more sophisticated than gold, Paula. Anyone can wear gold, but it takes someone like you to wear silver. Now isn't nice jewelry much better than some silly old doll?"

I didn't reply, but I could feel the weight of disappointment well within me. There were still packages left to open, but none big enough to be a Tiny Tears doll. We looked at the pictures in the Nancy Drew books, and smelled our perfume and dusting powder. Then my mother drew out a slender box and handed it to my sister.

"Sharon, this is for you. I had it specially made."

Inside was a dainty gold watch.

"That was my watch. It's real gold. And that band is just right for you; it belongs on a delicate wrist. Paula could never wear something like that, could you, Paula?" And she got up and left the room.

I hung my head in shame and rage. Why hadn't I gotten a special gift, and why couldn't I wear pretty things, too? Could I help it that I was already five inches taller than my mother, and an inch taller than my sister? I hated the watch, and I hated Sharon.

Then I heard something rattling in the hall. Mother entered, carrying a large box wrapped in Santa Claus paper.

"Here, you baby, this is for you," she said, and pushed the box to me across the carpeting.

I tore at the paper excitedly. It was just what I wanted! Tiny Tears and her layette, just the one I had seen at Hudson's.

I jumped up, ran to my mother, and gave her a big hug.

"Thank your father, too. I bought the doll, but after all, he pays the bills around here."

I gave my dad a quick hug, then turned to take Tiny Tears gently from her box. It was the best Christmas ever.

Tiny Tears was wonderful, perhaps the best gift I had ever received from my parents. Tiny Tears could drink and wet, and she kept me busy feeding and changing her.

I played with the doll endlessly, feeding her, rocking her, carrying her from room to room with me, changing her diaper and clothes, giving her baths, reading to her, putting her to bed for a nap, and then waking her up again. There was just one little dark spot clouding my happiness. Finally, after many days of agonizing thought, I got up my nerve and went hesitantly to my mother.

"Please don't tell my girlfriends that I got a doll for Christmas. They'd laugh at me."

"Oh, yeah?" My mother looked interested. "Well, I thought it was dumb to give somebody your age a doll, but I finally decided to get one for you so you'd stop pestering me and maybe get those stupid baby dolls out of your system."

I played with Tiny Tears endlessly from December to my birthday in March, sleeping with her, cradling her, bathing her, singing to her. Sometimes my mother would be pleased with my happiness, and say so. But mostly she'd say, "Paula, you're still a baby," shake her head and walk away.

Then it was my twelfth birthday. My mother gave me my first nylons and a garter belt and a pale green polished cotton shirt-waist with embroidered flowers that was the most beautiful dress I'd ever seen. Mother had baked me a pink heart cake with pale pink, cinnamon-flavored icing, and my best friend Susan was spending the day. What a great birthday!

We were running, pink cheeked, from the basement to my room, where I had carefully hidden Tiny Tears under my bed just before Susan arrived, when we stopped to get a drink of water in the kitchen.

"Paula, did you show Susan your new dress and your nylon stockings?" I nodded yes. "You girls are getting all grown up. Just imagine, 12! It's time to give up your baby toys."

"Baby toys?" Susan wrinkled her nose and looked at me. I could feel myself starting to blush. "What do you mean by baby toys, Mrs. Miner?"

"Paula knows what I mean, Susan, don't you, Paula?"

I looked down at my hands and didn't answer.

"Do you still play with dolls, Susan?"

"Dolls? No, not since I was 9 or 10."

"Do you know what? Paula still plays with dolls. She even got a great big baby doll--a Tiny Tears--for Christmas. She plays with it constantly. She even sleeps with it."

Susan and my mother looked at each other and burst out laughing.

That night, I pulled Tiny Tears out from under my bed. I wiped her face tenderly, adjusted her clothes, looked over her layette, and then packed her away in the attic.

I never played with Tiny Tears--or any doll--again.

Chapter 13

Broom Dance

As she grew older, my best friend, Susan became more and more beautiful. She had dark brown hair and hazel eyes and an alabaster complexion, dimples, and a wonderful personality. She knew how to charm, how to flirt, how to converse. She had boyfriends, boys who would walk her home from grade school, carry her books, hold her hand, snatch a kiss.

In fact, all of the girls in our little club had boyfriends; all, except me. I was taller than most of the boys in the class, and so they never chose me as a dancing partner in gym class or at grade school dances. My parents had convinced me early and often of my big nose, buck teeth and receding chin. Of course I believed them; father knew best--so did mother. I turned their ridicule in on myself. I would look in the mirror and see the ugliness and understand why the boys didn't like me. My self-hatred deepened.

There was a new horror show on television Friday nights about this time, hosted by a creature named Morgus who had a hump back, huge teeth, shaggy hair and dark circles around his eyes. He lived in an ice house on the Detroit River.

The first time we watched this as a family and my dad saw the host, he said, "Hey Paula, there's your double. Morgus. Doesn't she look like Morgus?" Everyone agreed. And so that is who I became to them--Morgus.

If I laughed about something at the dinner table, Mother or Dad would say, "Close your mouth, Morgus, your fangs are hanging out," and then they'd laugh. Or, "Straighten up, Morgus, your hump is showing." Sometimes I would laugh with them, feeling that negative attention is better than none. Still, inside, I hurt.

I would try, sometimes, to talk to my mother about my lack of popularity with boys. She often seemed concerned if I was feeling blue.

"Why don't you play the piano? That always makes you feel better, or take a walk."

But I hung about the kitchen sighing deeply, not knowing how to broach the subject, until finally, I would allow it to tumble out.

"Everybody has a boyfriend but me!" Or, "The other night at Joanne's party there was one girl too many and someone had to dance with the broom."

"Dance with a broom?" My mother paused in her apple pie making to look me in the face.

"Yeah. Joanne kept one real dim light on and we were supposed to tap each other and change partners, but they just danced with their boyfriends and kept shoving the broom at me."

"So you went to your first boy-girl party and danced with a broom?"

"Well, only for a little while, and then I just let the thing fall on the floor and I went and sat down."

"In the dark? You were sitting there alone in the dark?"

"Well, yeah, because none of the boys would dance with me. And then they all stopped dancing and nobody was saying anything for a long time and then Joanne's mother put the light on and all the boys and girls were making out. So then we had to leave."

"Well, I'm sorry you had such a terrible time, Paula. But don't worry, those boys will grow. You'll be in high school in January and there will be lots of tall boys then, all kinds of boys for you to choose from, and you won't give those shrimps from Isaac Newton another thought."

It felt so good when I had those private little talks with my mother. She seemed to know so much and to be able to make me feel better, and I said so before I left the kitchen.

I went to the living room to play the piano until Dad got home. I heard his car, and the side door close, and then, just as I was finishing the piece, his deep laugh rose up, mingled with my mother's, and floated out of the kitchen.

Amid their laughter I heard the word "broom."

Chapter 14

The Rec Room

It was the era of the recreation room, and Dad had constructed ours downstairs. He built bookshelves on three walls to house his enormous collection of hardcovers and paperbacks, paneled the other walls, built a brick fireplace equipped with an outlet to accommodate gas logs, and tiled the floors.

We bought new furniture--Danish Modern was all the rage--and one of those portable televisions that everyone else had gotten two years earlier when they first came in vogue.

"Where did you get the paneling? It looks cheap," Mother told Dad as he drove in the last nails. "And that fireplace. Whoever heard of a fireplace out of cinder blocks? You should have used brick. At least that would have matched the paneling and the floor. Cinder blocks! I'm telling you."

Dad stood looking at the floor, the hammer hanging loosely from his fingers as Mother walked away, shaking her head.

Sharon and I each took hold of one of his hands.

"It's okay, Daddy," Sharon whispered. "We like the rec room. It's wonderful!"

"Yeah, Daddy," I added. "And the fireplace! Can we build a fire now?"

Dad shook his head.

"Nope. It's a fake fireplace. You have to buy pretend logs."

"When can we get some, Daddy? Will we buy them with Green Stamps?"

"Nope, no logs. Nothing. There isn't going to be a fireplace."

And with that, he collected his tools, put them away in the furnace room, and went upstairs.

The gas fireplace was important for it would have provided heat for that cold corner of the basement. Still, Mother, Sharon and I used the rec room every night and all day each Sunday, when we would bundle up in quilts to watch old movies on television, while Dad remained upstairs, reading, doing crossword puzzles or working in the garden.

He never once sat with us in the rec room to read or watch television. In fact, he only sat on the Danish modern couch in the mornings to lace up his heavy construction boots and in the evenings to remove them after work.

Mother frequently mentioned the mud.

Chapter 15

What the Animals Said

I stood at the side door and watched as the grey clouds disappeared in wisps and the sun broke through. The rain, a deep, drenching, mud-making rain had poured down on Detroit for days.

I was normally a lover of rain and the tiny iridescent puddles they brought where I would launch maple tree airplanes by the dozens. But I resented this rain. It took too long to be over. It kept me from my father's beloved yard where, adorned in daisy and clover chains and with dandelion smeared on my nose as proof that I liked butter, I reigned supreme over the robins and the worms they pulled, over the dazzling perennial beds, over the myriad annuals--portulaca, petunia, marigold, salvia--that grew everywhere under my father's loving touch.

I stood at the side door looking out, breathing my hot breath onto the window and making fingerprint faces which I quickly erased with the curtain so that Mother did not see me dirtying the glass.

While I traced the claw and teeth marks that our Airedale, Vicky had chewed in the door, I whined to my mother in the kitchen. "The sun's finally out! Can I play outside now?"

"No. It's muddy out there, and you'll track mud all over the house."

"But, please, Mother? I'll be careful. I'll stay on the sidewalk. I promise! And I won't step in a single puddle."

"No. I said no. You'll have to wait inside until the sun has time to dry things out. You can wait."

"For how long? How long will it take?"

"I don't know, an hour, maybe two. Not long."

"Two hours! That's too long. Please let me go out now, just for a few minutes? I want to see the raindrops on the rose petals. Please, Mother? I'll be good."

"Well, all right. But remember what I said--"

I was already out the door, my mother's last words still in the house. I ran to the old apple tree abloom in the yard and hugged its twisted brown trunk. Then I grabbed one of the sturdy branches and shook it gently, giggling at the miniature shower of petals and rain.

I stopped to touch the horns on a snail ambling along the sidewalk, but it shrank into its shell, so I went to watch the families of big black ants scurry over the fragrant peonies which they never harmed but seemed always to enjoy in great numbers.

I skated through the wet grass, my legs spattered with mud, until I reached the rose bed just below my bedroom window. There, I said hello to each of my friends in turn, the deeply perfumed red roses, the peace rose, and my favorites, the pink roses. I blew at the raindrops that shimmered in the velvet bowls, tracing the buds that had appeared from out of the storm with a tiny, gentle finger.

Suddenly, I felt something tickle my hand. There was a spider on my dress! I screamed and ran for the house, shouting over and over again for my mother, and holding my skirt out in front of me.

She opened the side door.

"What's wrong? Are you hurt? Did you fall?" She shouted her questions over my cries.

"A spider!" I screamed. "There's a spider on my dress. Get it off! Please get it off of me!"

She quickly knelt down and slipped her arm around my waist. With her free hand, she picked off the plump white spider and tossed it in the begonias near the door.

"There. It's gone. It's all better now. Are you all right?"

I shook my head yes. She gave me a hug and helped dry my eyes. Then she sat me on her lap in the kitchen.

"Poor little Paula. You like snails and crickets and ladybugs. Even the bees don't bother you. Now, why don't you like spiders?"

"They have too many legs and they look all fat and full of pus. And this one scared me because it jumped right off a rose and onto my dress." I shivered.

Mother rested her chin on my head.

"Do you know why the spider jumped on your dress? No? Well, it's because all of the trees and the flowers and the birds and the bugs talk to each other in the garden. And do you know what they say?"

I waited, wide-eyed, for my mother to tell me.

"They all talk about their favorite little friend--I heard them just last week-- how she helps to plant and water the flowers and feed the birds and she rescues ladybugs from the house and shoos the flies out when they get locked indoors.

"The spiders all came and listened very carefully for the name of the person who wouldn't step on them. And do you know whose name they heard?"

"Whose?"

"Yours. They said, 'Whenever we need a friend, Paula is there for us. She'll help you too, Mr. Spider.' And that's why the spider jumped on your dress. So that you could be his friend."

And Mother smiled down at me.

Chapter 16

Nightmares

The dream was always the same--a blond man crouched behind the bushes, behind the door, beside my bed. As I began to scream, he would rise and creep toward me, a knife in his hand.

I jumped out of bed and ran to my parents' room. They hadn't heard my screams. I shook my dad's shoulder gently. He snorted, and when I shook him again, he woke up.

"Who is it? Paula?"

"It's me, Dad," I whispered.

"Who's there? What's wrong?" Now my mother was awake, too.

"I'm scared," I said. "There's someone in my room. That man." I looked over my shoulder into the darkness.

"There's no one there. You had that dream again. Go back to bed and let us get our rest." My mother sounded disgusted.

I did not move, but started crying, softly.

Mother groaned.

"Go ahead, Paul. You go with her this time. Lie down with her until she falls asleep."

Chapter 17

The Conversation

For a long time, until Sharon was graduated from Isaac Newton School and went on to high school, we would walk the ten blocks home for lunch, have 20 minutes in which to eat, then hurry back to school in the afternoon.

Mother would often have wonderful surprises waiting for our noon meal--homemade potato pancakes with sour cream; bacon, lettuce and tomato sandwiches with mayo on white bread so soft your fingerprints stayed in it; chicken gumbo soup and cream cheese spread on bread.

But on this particular day when we came in the side door, there was no food warming on the stove, the table had not been laid for lunch and Mother was not in the kitchen.

"Mother? Mother!"

No answer.

"Mother!" Sharon's voice rang down the basement stairs.

Strange, muffled noises came from the rear of the house. We ran down the hall to our bedroom. Mother's backside was sticking out of the closet. From time to time her hand, holding a rag, would appear, dip into the bucket of graying, soapy water, then disappear into the closet again as she scrubbed the hardwood floor.

As she brought the wet cloth out of the bucket, the dirty water sloshed over the top of my new box of paper dolls, and ran down the sides in small trickles that wet our Monopoly game.

"Mother! Mother? What are you doing?"

There was no reply.

"You're getting our things all wet!"

"Then move all that crap out of the way. You just threw it into the closet. Why are you so worried about it now?"

Sharon and I hurried to move the pile of shoes, stuffed animals, dolls and games. Mother continued scrubbing. Occasionally we heard snatches of her muffled muttering: "Damned little jerks..." "Never any help..." "Get shit and shoved in it..." "A prison around here..."

Finally she backed all the way out of the closet, stood up and glared at us.

"You little devils," she said, waving her finger, her face tight with rage, "you two little devils and that father of yours will be the death of me. I'm going to get myself a job and get the hell out of here. Then you'll never see me again!"

"No Mother, no, don't leave us. Please don't leave us! We're sorry! We won't do it again!" Sharon wailed.

"What did we do wrong, Mother, why are you mad? Please don't go away and leave us." By this time I, too, was crying.

"Well if I don't leave, you will! Something's got to give. I'll send you two to the orphanage--to Auntie Annie's!"

"No, Mama! Please don't send us there," Sharon pleaded, sobbing. "We'll be good! We'll be good."

Suddenly the phone, which sat in a small alcove between the two bedrooms, began to ring.

Mother cleared her throat angrily.

As she stepped on our toys to get to the phone, she slipped in a wet spot and kicked over a large metal can. Marbles bounced out and spilled everywhere, rolling under the beds and the dresser and smacking against the walls.

" Damn it! That's all I need!" she shouted.

"It's okay, Mother," Sharon said as she began to scramble about. "We'll pick them up. What about lunch?"

"Lunch? You expect me to make you lunch after all I've done for you today? Slap some peanut butter on a piece of bread and then get the hell out of here, or you'll be late for school."

Fearful of having to pass by Mother on her way to the bathroom for clean tissue, Sharon took two used Kleenexes out of her pocket and handed one of them to me. We dried our eyes, blew our noses and began picking up the marbles as quietly as possible so we wouldn't disturb our mother.

"Hello? Oh, hello, Annie. How are you?"

Sharon and I looked at each other in fear. Auntie Annie!

Mother would tell what happened and then our aunt would come and take us away!

Sure enough, as we listened, our mother described the scene that had just taken place, how she never had help with us or the house, how she never saw our father who was always busy with a remodeling project or at work in the garden after supper.

"Just at meals. Otherwise I never see him. He has nothing to do with me. I'm just his chief cook and bottle washer and that's it."

Auntie Annie made some reply.

Mother was crying now.

"Uh. Uh. Never. Not since the operation. Can you believe it? That was two years ago! He said the men at work told him after that kind of operation, it would be like using a paper bag.

"He hasn't touched me since."

My aunt said something else.

"Who knows? Eh! Who cares? He goes to those union meetings once a week. They probably have whores there for him to use."

Mother was crying harder now. Sharon ran to get her a Kleenex from the bathroom, and Mother wiped her eyes and pressed the tissue to her nose.

"Annie, can I call you later? If I don't make some lunch for the girls right now, they'll be late getting back to school."

Mother hung up and sat on her bed, looking off into the distance. The telephone was still in her lap.

"Do you want me to put the phone back for you, Mother?" I asked hesitantly, afraid that if I spoke, she would start yelling again.

"What? No, I'll do it."

Mother looked at us and sighed.

"Come here you two poor little kids."

She held out her arms to us and then squeezed us tightly as we crowded around her. "I'm sorry I got so angry. Now you'll be upset for school and it will be all my fault. Girls, don't worry about those marbles. I'll pick up the rest. Just keep your closet nice and clean and orderly from now on, O.K.? Now, let's go make some lunch."

Chapter 18

Grand Mal

About two years after her hysterectomy, about the time that my sister's epileptic seizures became more frequent and more intense, Mother left home to go to work part time making price tags on an IBM machine in the marking department at the J.L. Hudson Company store miles away.

She became a fulltime employee, and left me in charge of the house--and my epileptic older sister. Apparently the doctor had trouble finding just the right dosage of Dilantin and phenobarbital to control Sharon's seizures for they were frequent and, of course, unpredictable.

Sharon had her first epileptic seizure on Palm Sunday during the service at Alpha Baptist Church in Detroit when she was seven. Pastor Hamm had just invited sinners to come forward, and the congregation was singing "Jesus Calls Us O'er the Tumult," when Sharon fell toward Dad. He managed to catch her by the dress just before her head hit the pew.

"Pull her dress down, Paul, pull her dress down, " my mother hissed at him. "Her panties are showing."

We were making our way down the aisle to the back of the church. My mother dabbed at her eyes with an embroidered hanky and my dad looked stiff and frightened.

"Mommy, what's wrong with Sharon?"

"Shh! Quiet. Don't ask so many questions. We don't know what's wrong with her. She just fainted, that's all."

By the time we reached the cool privacy of the pastor's study,

Sharon was conscious. She drank some water that one of the deacons brought and then we left. At home my parents tried to find out what Sharon remembered of the incident.

"What happened to you, Sharon? Do you know what happened? How did you feel just before you fainted?"

But Sharon was too young. She could recall getting dizzy, nothing more. The next day, mother took Sharon to the doctor. After examining her he concluded that she must have a virus and said she should stay home a day or two to be on the safe side.

"What should I write in her excuse to the school? Do I have to tell what happened?"

"Just write that she had the flu. That will be good enough. That's probably what it is, anyway," the doctor said.

At home, Sharon and I were reminded again and again not to say anything at school about the "fainting spells." Mother insisted on the term that would conceal Sharon's illness, that would shield her from the status of invalid or the stigma of mental retardation that seemed to prevail at home. So great was the secrecy surrounding Sharon's epilepsy that I was forbidden to telephone a neighbor should she have a seizure when my sister and I were alone. Mother and Dad lived in fear of their jobs--or pretended to--so that we were never allowed to call them at work if a problem arose at home. Never mind the sitters. After I turned seven and Sharon was nine and a half, my parents decided that we were old enough to handle things on our own.

"You're too old for babysitters," Mother would say. "Just remember to keep the doors locked and you'll be fine. After all, you have each other."

What we didn't have, though, was an adult to call in emergencies. I had asked, even begged to be able to call the next door neighbor for help.

"We don't want any busybodies in the neighborhood knowing our business," she replied. "Why do you think we got off the partyline and arranged for an unlisted phone number?"

"But she's nice. She's our friend, not a busybody. And besides, she already knows," I replied. "Don't you remember that time on the bus when we were bringing Sharon back from the doctor's after one of her spells? You talked with Mrs. Grant all the way home."

Mother thought hard for a minute.

"Oh, that. O.K. I remember. She thinks it's allergies. I told Mrs. Grant Sharon sometimes has bad allergic reactions, and she believed me. So don't you go telling her otherwise. You don't want her to think that you're a liar, do you?"

One winter day when Sharon was 12 and I was 10, we were sitting on her bed playing "Go to the Head of the Class" when she suddenly began having what I now know was a Grand Mal seizure. I grabbed the game board, set it out of the way, pulled Sharon back onto her bed, and managed to stick a corner of the bedspread between her teeth before she bit her lips and tongue. So severe were her convulsions that the only way I could keep her from falling off the bed was to brace my feet against my bed, wedge my hands under her mattress, and lay across her chest.

I remained that way for 20 minutes, crying and praying for the seizure to end.

When it finally did, I ran to the bathroom for a towel and wastebasket and stood sobbing, waiting for Sharon to throw up, which she invariably did as she regained consciousness.

This time, though, she was slow to come around. I debated, watching her, listening to see if she was still breathing. I decided to chance it. I called the office from which my father was sent each day to a construction site in the Detroit area where he was needed as a pipefitter. The secretary said he was somewhere in the city, driving from one job assignment to another.

"Will you please have him come home when you find him?" I sobbed into the phone. "Just tell him his oldest daughter is real sick."

Then I did the unthinkable once again. I called my mother at work. In the several minutes it took her to come to the phone, I picked at the cuticles on my thumb and forefinger until they bled.

"Mother?" My voice trembled. "I'm sorry to bother you, but Sharon's real sick. Can you come home now? Please? I'm scared she might die or something."

"Aw, you're nuts. She's not going to die. Grow up, Paula, and quit bothering me. Stop always thinking of yourself and your problems and start thinking of others. Be a Christian, Paula. You know how to take care of her. Just do it. I can't leave here for another hour, and besides, how would I get home? I don't have a car. I don't even drive!"

"Please, Mother! Can't you take a cab? Just this once? I'm scared. Sharon had a real bad spell!"

"No. And quit bothering me at work or you're going to get it when I get home. Now go. Go on and take care of Sharon. After all, you are her sister!"

As I returned to the bedroom, Sharon was coming to. I was holding the wastebasket while she vomited when Dad hurried in.

"What's going on? Why did you call?"

"Sharon was real bad this time and I got scared."

Dad took the wastebasket, emptied it, and washed it out. When he returned, he put a cold cloth on Sharon's forehead and covered her.

"Just stay here and watch her until Mother and I get home. She'll probably sleep all night now, but don't leave this room, just in case. And don't call me at work any more when Sharon gets this way. You can handle it, Paula; that's what you're here for--to help others."

Chapter 19

Doing Dishes

I heard my mother as I descended the stairs. She was swearing to herself in the laundry-kitchen area where we cooked and ate in the summer when it was hot. We had another complete kitchen down there, an old granite-top table and black steel chairs with black covers. The table had a drawer in it with eight place settings of old silverplate that Mother moved downstairs when we got the Oneida Wear with S & H Green Stamps.

I walked down slowly and quietly in my Indian slippers, wanting to be quiet so my mother wouldn't yell at me.

"What's wrong, Mother? Why are you mad?"

"Eh! I have so much to do around this stupid house, I hate it. Never get any help but do something wrong and you get shit and shoved in it!"

All the lights were on and she was standing in front of one of the cupboards that contained three complete sets of dishes--dishes with blue flowers collected from boxes of oatmeal, Fiesta Ware plates, cups and saucers, bowls and salt and pepper shakers, and a set of everyday china decorated with red and yellow tulips.

"Look at all this crap! Why the hell is he always buying me dishes? I need new clothes, some nice perfume, something special for a woman, but no! He buys me dishes. It makes me so mad I could scream. When are we ever going to use any of this crap? I'm so damned mad right now I could scream!"

And she cleared her throat hard as she always did when she was angry.

"We need to get rid of some of this crap, but I want to do it now, not wait for those bums from the Goodwill to come and pick the stuff up. I hate to have them in the house, the way they look at you. Probably looking around for stuff to steal and murder you to boot, or worse! I'm going to get rid of this stuff myself, right now."

She went to the furnace room where Dad's tools were mounted neatly on the red walls and returned with a big hammer. She dragged one of the kitchen chairs to the cupboard, took down a stack of dishes, set them in the deep laundry tub and started hitting them, cracking them, smashing them into tiny pieces with every blow of her hammer. I was frightened and felt like crying. Why was she acting like this, why was she breaking all the beautiful dishes?

Suddenly she threw her head back and laughed wildly. She couldn't stop. As she laughed she looked at me, her eyes filling.

"You think I'm crazy, don't you? You think I'm nuts! Well, if I am, it's all of your fault; you, your sister's, your dad's. Always giving, never getting shit in return! I've had it!"

More shards flew up as Mother swung the hammer harder. Suddenly, she thrust it at me.

"Here! Do you want try it?"

She was still laughing, offering me the hammer. I was horrified, bewildered. We were always spanked, even for so much as spilling a glass of milk. It was a much greater offense to break something when we set the table or did the dishes. I wanted to break dishes with a hammer, too. It looked like so much fun. But wouldn't I be punished?

"What if Daddy finds out? He gave them to you."

"Well he's bound to, and so what if he does find out! What could he do about it after they're all broken? Anyway, we can hide them. I'll put the pieces in a big brown paper bag and you can take them to the alley. Just put them way down in the garbage can.

" But he may look."

"You can hide them in the neighbor's garbage cans. Just make sure they don't see you. Anyway, it's fun to break these damn things. Here, go ahead. Don't be afraid, I'll protect you, just like I always do."

"But what if he comes home and catches us?"

"He won't. It's only," Mother squinted over her shoulder at the teapot clock on the wall. "It's only two o'clock. He won't be home until 4:30. Are you scared?"

I nodded.

"Here, come here, honey."

Mother put her arm around my shoulder and her hand over mine on the hammer. Whack! I watched in fascination as our blow broke the dinner plates into thirds.

I giggled and looked up at Mother. She smiled down at me. I felt a rush of love.

"How about a nice cup and saucer? Here's a big fat orange cup and a dark blue saucer. Aren't these ugly colors? I always hated this Fiesta crap. Always. Daddy's mother gave it to us. Here. Go ahead."

The large chunks that rolled and scattered in the wash tub reminded me of the night sky in my favorite picture book.

"Shh! Wait a minute! I hear something."

As we stopped to listen, the side door slammed shut.

"Mother! Daddy's home! He's going to catch us!"

"Shh! Quiet. Paul? Is that you, dear?"

Mother moved swiftly to the doorway.

"No, don't come down, it's all wet down here. I just finished waxing the floor. What did you want? Well, go ahead and use the bathroom upstairs.... No, it's all right. I haven't cleaned it yet. I was going to do that while the wax dries, so go ahead. Come on, Paula. Let's go upstairs now. She's a good helper, aren't you, Paula. She helped me wax the floor, Dad."

Mother rolled her eyes at me, let out a ragged breath, and together, we climbed the stairs. Later, I carried the broken dishes out in heavy paper sacks and distributed them in garbage cans up and down the alley.

When Dad asked two weeks later, Mother told him she had donated the dishes to the poor people who came by in the big Goodwill truck. Spring cleaning and doing good, she said, often go hand in hand.

Chapter 20

Desserts

Dad pushed his chair back from the table. It made a scaping sound on the linoleum.

"I'm going to weed some more before it gets dark." He belched loudly and stood up. "Thank you all for dinner."

"Why don't you stay in here with us for once, instead of always running outside right away?" Mother spoke without turning around.

"And do what?"

The screen door shut behind him.

My mother, Sharon and I continued to sit at the kitchen table, trying to ignore the heat of early August.

"Would you like tea with milk and sugar, anyone? You know how good it tastes with candy bars."

Each of us usually had a candy bar for dessert. It was Tuesday, and my dad didn't do the grocery shopping until Wednesday night, so there were only three candy bars left from the three packages of six bars each that he purchased the week before: a Mr. Goodbar; a Heath Bar and a milk chocolate Nestle's bar. Both Sharon and I wanted the Nestle's.

"Oh, let Sharon have the Nestle's, Paula. You like nuts, have the Mr. Goodbar; I'm having the Heath."

"But Sharon always gets to pick. I want the Nestle's this time."

"I'll have Dad buy another box of Nestle's tomorrow night. You can wait one day, can't you? Besides, I think you ate most of those Nestle bars anyway, didn't you?"

"I did not! Sharon did! You know she dosen't like candy with nuts, and she only likes a Heath bar once in awhile!"

"Yeah? That's what you say, but I know different."

"Ask Sharon. Isn't it true, Sharon, you don't like candy with nuts!"

Before my sister could reply, Mother interrupted. "Stop trying to make a liar out of me, Paula. Anyway, I think you've snuck out of bed once in awhile late at night and taken an extra one, or there would be more left."

"I didn't, Mother, and I want the Nestle bar," I protested, beginning to cry at her betrayal. "You always make me give in to Sharon."

"Well, I want Sharon to have the Nestle's bar tonight. Go ahead, you can get them, Sharon, and give me the Heath. Besides, Paula, aren't you going over to Susan's house tomorrow for the day? Sharon never gets to do anything special because of her problem, so you should give in to her once in awhile. She never gets anything special. One lousy candy bar and you're making such a big deal out of it!"

Sharon had sat silently, leafing through a Seventeen Magazine, oblivious to the battle at the table. From time to time she tore a strip of paper off a larger sheet to mark a page and make a notation on a scratch pad.

"Paula, Sharon's busy. She wants to show me some things that she'd like to get for her birthday. Will you get the candy bars? Please, Paula. I'm so tired from being on my feet all day I can hardly stand up. And get yourself a Kleenex and blow your nose. You need to save those tears for something important instead of crying over a stupid candy bar. There'll be worse times ahead. Just you wait. You'll need them then."

Still crying, I fetched the candy bars, then sat at the table to eat the Mr. Goodbar.

"What did you want to show me, Sugar Plum?"

Sharon was almost through with a Glamour Magazine. She said, "I've made a list for my birthday, and I wanted to show you a few things that you can buy at Hudson's."

"More things, Sharon? Always wanting something. Not like my poor Paula, here, never asking for a thing, do you, Paula? Well, you're a good girl not to drain your poor old ma of her last nickel."

Before I could reply, Mother and Sharon had their heads together, looking at the pages that Sharon had marked. Because Sharon's birthday was in late summer, she usually received things to wear beyond the requisite school clothes that replaced those we had outgrown.

Sharon always had beautiful taste in clothes, going for the traditional rather than offbeat fashions that would go out of style quickly, and she and Mother oohed and ahed over the pleated wool skirts in rich plaids and russets and golds, over the soft, bulky Angora sweaters from Italy, over the leather flats and loafers and the fine leather purses and the chain necklaces, bracelets and belts that were splashed across the pages.

"My! Don't they have beautiful things this year!"

"They do, Mother," Sharon said excitedly. Consulting her scratch pad, she flipped to the back pages in the "Where to Buy" section and began showing the items that could be purchased at Hudson's. "Look, Mother, isn't this great? You can get me what I want for my birthday and use your discount at Hudson's to do it!"

"Yes, I suppose I can."

Mother pushed back her chair and began clearing the dinner table. She stacked the dirty dishes in the sink. Then she looked out into the yard as she rinsed them in hot water.

"Look at him, always outside, groveling in the dirt like some peasant instead of spending a little time in here with us. Damn it anyway! I just get the darn charge paid off and something else comes along! And your father will never fork over the money to help. That's why I had to go to work. He's still mad about it two years later. But I just had to get a job in order to get you kids and myself a few nice things. If it were up to him, we'd all be sitting here wearing rags, he's so damned tight with his money.

"But it's not so bad with my dear little Paula to help me so much at home. You're a good helper, aren't you, Paula? And never asking for anything! How could I be so lucky to get such a considerate, thoughtful daughter who is so unselfish? Never thinks of herself, always helping others! Paula, someday God's going to give you a diamond crown!"

Chapter 21

The Grim Precinct

Right now I am struggling to perform more than one or two tasks a day, say, teaching my classes, driving the children to school, or washing a few dishes. I find grocery shopping difficult and somehow emotionally painful, perhaps because at these suicidal times when I am feeling so very worthless, I do not want to engage in any activity that is life-sustaining.

I am lethargic. There is a heaviness in my limbs, sometimes an ache with infrequent, unlocalized, shooting pains throughout my body that always make me wonder if I am developing the rheumatoid arthritis that has crippled my mother.

And sometimes a sudden and horrible tingling begins in the top of my head, as if my scalp were on fire. This sensation often moves down the middle of my skull to the base of my neck and across to the left behind my ear, where it turns into a dull, throbbing ache. I frequently feel a burning sensation in my eyes, and a heaviness in my eyelids. I often have dark circles under my eyes.

I crave sweets, and sour foods such as plain yogurt, during these depressed periods, tastes sour to me. At other times, I lose my appetite.

I am unable to stay warm. Even in summer, I often get chilled and use four or five blankets, two of them 100 percent wool.

There is an extreme and constant heaviness in my chest that makes breathing difficult. I contract frequent upper respiratory infections that are either brought on by some mechanism of depression that weakens my immune system, or that, themselves, bring on severe depression. It's a chicken-egg problem: do I first get severely depressed, and then become physically ill, or do I get sick, and then severely depressed?

Of course, there is the unrelenting desire to sleep. When I give in to this desire, my sleep is dead, dreamless. Yet I awaken exhausted.

I'm frustrated at the things around me that need to be done and at my inability to do them, so I become angry at my slatternly self. No cheerful inner dialogue, no stern self-rebuke can bring me out of this. On the one hand, I feel victimized by thoughts of suicide, and on the other, I am half in love with easeful death. There is a shadow on my soul.

My thoughts are confused and I suffer considerable memory loss. I can't remember what it was that I had planned to do just a few minutes before. I often suffer a vague sense of paranoia, that I'm not doing my work adequately, that I'm not meeting my children's needs.

I have a deep desire to help myself out of this feeling of victimization -- clinically depressed people do not want to be this way. But because the suffering of the clinically depressed is often lifelong, we do not know that the way we feel is abnormal. For us, the lightness that comes with a true joy for living may surface periodically, seasonally, rarely, or sadly, not at all.

I had been treated for depression in the 1970s by a psychiatrist whose aim it was to find the proper medication, put me on it, then check with me from time to time to see how I was doing. I hated the medicine that dried out my body from my mouth to my bowels, adding to my discomfort instead of relieving it.

I also resented having to be dependant upon medication for something I believed at the time to be strictly psychological. So about six or eight months after I began the regimen, I flushed the pills down the toilet and decided to go it alone.

Nothing changed through the years. The depression, the anger, the frustration, the guilt stayed with me, and so did the frequent upper respiratory infections, which I was developing now, both summer and winter instead of just in cold weather.

As an over-achiever ever striving to win the approval of my parents, I got my Ph.D. and a job teaching journalism and English at a small college in Michigan where there was a wonderful, motherly secretary named Jeannette Leahy. She cared about me and about how I was feeling, and I felt embarassed that my reports were always so negative. Imagine my elation when, one freezing cold day full of sunshine that made the heaps of snow glisten and glitter, I came in excitedly to work to tell Jeannette how wonderful I felt, that I could never remember having been this way before. I was actually happy! The heaviness in my chest was gone--I could breathe! I was all lightness and air and felt as if I were floating.

"This is how others feel," I remember saying. "This is how it feels to be normal and not depressed. I've finally broken through!"

The feeling lasted one whole day. The next morning, when I awoke, the lethargy had returned. Yet that single day became a benchmark at which to aim. It gave me the hope that one day, I might feel that way again.

Chapter 22

The Ghost of Uncle John

In Detroit that glorious day in early spring, the fierce rain over night had stopped and the trees, that gentle, shining morning, were putting forth baby leaves that always made me think of tiny chartreuse hands reaching toward the sky.

"Paula? It's Pam!"

"Pam! Hello! I'm so glad you called! How are you? Where are you?"

"I'm home for Spring Break. Let's do something!"

"O.K. What?"

"Would you like to come over for lunch? Come right away if you can. We've got a lot to catch up on. We'll just sit and gab all day."

How long had it been since I had seen my dear cousin? I took a quick shower, got in the car and drove over. Pam and I talked all morning about college classes, boyfriends, politics, music, books. Sometime during lunch as Aunt Jen joined us and we sat munching tuna salad sandwiches, hardboiled eggs and chips, our conversation turned to our relatives --uncles, aunts, cousins--and how and what they were doing.

Finally, Pam said, "Doesn't it seem strange to you that you have three uncle Johns, while the rest of the people in the world usually only have one?"

"Two."

"Two what?"

"Two uncle Johns. I only have two, not three."

"Uh-huh. You have three."

"My dear Pam, I ought to know how many uncle Johns I have, oughtn't I? I have two: Uncle John, my dad's brother in Chicago, and Uncle John, Dad's brother-in-law in Detroit. See? Two uncle Johns."

"What about our mothers' brother John? You're forgetting him."

"That's because he dosen't exist."

Pam and Aunt Jen looked at each other.

"Yes, he does, Paula," Pam said evenly. "You know, our mothers' brother-- John."

"What? What are you guys talking about?" I looked from Pam to Aunt Jen. "You're fooling me! I've never heard of him. There is no such person."

"Yes, there is, Paula," Aunt Jen said. There was no hint of laughter in her voice. "He's our little brother; Johnny is Grandpa and Grandma's last child."

"But Mother always called you the baby," I protested to Aunt Jen.

"Well, I'm not. Johnny is the last. He's why Grandpa and Grandma stopped having children."

"Where is he?"

"Up North in Lapeer, Michigan. In a home. He'll be there the rest of his life."

"Why? What's wrong with him?"

"A lot of things. He's retarded, for one, and then he got to be a teenager, bigger and stronger than Grandpa. He couldn't handle Johnny any more. So they put him away."

"Does Mother know about him?"

"Well, of course she does. She helped take care of him. She helped with all of us, being the oldest. Sure she knows. We all go to visit him together once in awhile."

"Why hasn't she ever told us about him?"

I don't know why, Paula. I'm surprised she hasn't; your dad knows about him. He's taken us there to visit Johnny. I don't know why she's never mentioned him to you. I just don't know."

I said nothing to my family about the conversation during dinner that night. But immediately after Dad had gone to bed and Mother was reading the paper in her chair in the living room, I whispered to Sharon that it was time. We sat down together on the couch and cleared our throats.

Mother looked from behind her paper at each of us.

"What are you two up to? What do you want?"

"We want to talk to you, don't we, Sharon?"

Sharon crossed her arms and nodded yes.

"That's right, Mother. We've come for a little chat. Paula and I would like a little information."

"Information? About what?"

"About your little brother John."

Sharon's words hung in the air like ice.

Mother cleared her throat. She glanced at her paper.

"I don't know what you're talking about. There is no John."

"Yes, there is, Mother. Aunt Jen and I had a very informative talk today. He came up quite by accident during our lunchtime conversation. Even Pam knows all about him. Why don't we?"

"Because there is no such person. They were fooling you, and you fell for it, you nut!"

"No, Mother, I'm not the nut, and neither is Sharon. But apparently you think that Uncle John--your baby brother-- is, or you wouldn't have kept him hidden from us all these years. Why did you, Mother? Are you ashamed of him? What's wrong with him, anyway?"

Mother crushed the paper in her lap.

"He's retarded, that's all. And he got too big to handle, so Grandpa had to put him away."

"Why didn't you ever tell us about him?"

"I just kept it to myself, that's all. I thought it would be best that way. You know how your dad always makes such fun of people. So I never said anything."

"You mean Dad doesen't know about this Uncle John, either?"

"No. And don't you go telling him!"

"Aunt Jen told me Dad has driven all of you to up to visit him in --let's see, now, what is the name of that place up North--ah, yes--Lapeer, where Sharon and I went that time to church camp--Lapeer, Michigan. Just think, Sharon!" I turned to my sister. "We had an uncle up there in Lapeer and didn't even know it. Why, I'm sure the Christians from the church camp would have been glad to take us for a visit to meet our long-lost uncle!"

We both stared at our Mother.

"Never mind, you two. See, here you go, making fun of poor Johnny. I just knew that this would happen. Now maybe you know why I never told you. I'm the oldest. It was my duty to protect him."

Chapter 23

Abuse, Abandonment and Love

Those of us who have been abused want to be loved, but we don't believe ourselves to be lovable. What we end up doing is searching for affection with a misguided sense of what love is. When we find it, it affirms the view that we are, in fact, no good. How does this happen? We look for companions who are exciting--or dangerous--and these harmful partners fulfill their role by repeating the patterns of abuse so customary, so normal to us. They oblige us by sending out the old familiar messages through their verbal, emotional, physical and sexual abuse: "See?" their words, their actions say. "It's true; you are unlovable, and that is why I am harming you."

Often the injury is psychic rather than physical; something--perhaps knowledge, or support, maybe trust, or even love--is withheld, thus giving the withholder a twisted sense of power. No matter what element is missing from the relationship, when it ends, the result is inevitably the same: there is an overwhelming sense of shame, worthlessness, and abandonment. Why have these patterns repeated themselves in my love relationships? Could it be familiarity? Could it be, ironically, that abandonment feels so horribly right because my own parents abandoned me over and over again in different ways throughout the years?

My mother abandoned me to my father who, while he never raped me, nonetheless abused me sexually. Her jokes to him about padded cells and shirts with straps were tantamount to tacit approval.

She abandoned me emotionally by teaching me with woodenspoon spankings and hard slaps across the face that the expression of anger is selfish and sinful. "You must learn to accept your lot in life, Paula, instead of always feeling sorry for yourself. It's God's plan for you."

She abandoned the family physically by removing herself from our home, by placing her own needs to escape the drudgery of housework and the confinement of a bad marriage above those of a physically ill daughter and one who became mentally and spiritually ill as the years progressed. She taught me early on that it is more blessed to give than to receive, then worked my neurotic personality to advantage--the more she took, the harder I tried to give--hoping against hope that somehow, I would win her love and approval.

The parental abandonment continued into my adult life. I was married and living in Toledo when my parents called to tell me their new address in Michigan--they had sold the house in which I grew up without ever telling me it was on the market. I never had the chance to say good-bye.

Then, when I was pregnant with Claire, ill with kidney problems and phlebitis and in desperate need of the love and understanding of a mother, I drove the 70 miles to their home in Southgate, looking for comfort and concern. Imagine my surprise when I walked into my parents' house one September Sunday just two weeks after a visit in August, and found everything in boxes and crates.

"What is this? Where are you going?"

"To Florida. We'll be leaving in three weeks," Mother said.

My eyes brimmed with tears.

"Moving? Why are you leaving? I need you so much right now."

Mother shrugged. "Nobody told you to have another kid. That's your problem. Dad and I just decided there's nothing here for us and it's time to leave. Oh, by the way, Paula, if you want any of that junk in the basement, you'd better look through it now. We're going to throw it all away before we leave."

Among the "junk" scattered about the basement floor was my baby book.

There was no emotional support when I got my divorce--whatever went wrong was undoubtedly my fault, according to my mother, who kept my former husband's photograph among the family pictures hanging in her hallway, but never thought to include one of me.

I have been frustrated in my attempts to discover the patterns in my parents' lives that have made them what they are. But my therapist in Nashville helped me to trace the patterns in my own upbringing that laid the dangerous foundations for adult relationships in which I was beaten, raped and abandoned emotionally over the years.

Not until I was able to understand the root causes of my self-loathing and to learn, little by little, to love my self, was I able to break those patterns of abuse and abandonment and begin meeting men and women who were genuine in their caring, their kindness, their love and their emotional support.

It is from these gentle people that I have learned how to live my life. I am grateful that I have been given that opportunity, but it did not come easily, or quickly.

Chapter 24

The Civics Lesson

I tied on my bathrobe, put on my slippers and wrapped myself in a quilt. I stood at the bottom of the basement stairs holding my pillow, a box of Kleenex and an absorbent bath towel.

"Mother?"

No answer.

"Mother?"

"Shh! Be quiet! What do you want now?"

"I just threw up again."

Mother did not answer right away. She was concentrating on the movie.

"Mother? I just threw up again."

She turned in her seat.

"Then what are you doing down here, you nut? I told you to stay upstairs if you're sick. Now go on, get going. You're spreading your germs all over the house. You've been sick with colds and flu for more than a month now. Every weekend, the same damn thing! Aren't you ever going to get better, Paula?"

I shook my head. The hot tears rolled down my cheeks and made wet spots on my pillow. I went over to a tall shelf and found a Nancy Drew book. I had stopped reading the series five years before.

"If you need something, call your father. He's up there doing nothing. Bother him for once. Go on now, get going."

I went slowly back upstairs. My father had fallen asleep over his book in the living room. I fixed my pillow against the headboard of my bed, climbed in, and pulled the covers up around me. I set "The Mystery of the Tolling Bell" beside me on the bed, and began cutting out the paper dolls that I'd had to beg my mother to buy. She had always bought me a coloring book and a set of paper dolls when I was a little girl if I got sick--something to keep me occupied when she had to work and left me alone.

But here I was, 15, and a sophomore at Cooley High School. I hadn't requested such a toy in two or three years. What had happened, she had wanted to know, to make me regress into childhood? I had shrugged. Maybe I was just tired of school. Maybe my Latin, honors English, biology, civics, vocal music and physical education classes were too difficult for me --I knew the geometry class was--I was flunking that, just as I had failed algebra the previous year. Maybe my mind just needed a break from homework, as my body did from housework, and all my systems had simply shut down.

A nasty flu had hit Detroit hard that winter, and I had caught it three times--a dubious kind of record among my friends. Even Susan, who suffered from asthma and bronchitis, had only had it twice. For me, the third bout was the charm. I stopped missing the toilet and puking on the rug, stopped having to wash the plastic waste basket out through bleary eyes and put away the heating pad that I had kept on my stomach to warm the vomit-sore muscles. This last time, the only remnant of flu was a deep, barking cough and thick yellow phlegm.

"You're not getting enough rest. Just finish the dinner dishes and then go to bed," Mother told me one evening.

"But I have a book report due in English and a civics test to study for," I protested hoarsely. "I can't go to bed yet."

Mother shrugged.

"Don't say I didn't warn you, Paula. If you don't get your rest, you'll get sicker and sicker, and then, good-bye! Now, what are you crying for? You have to take care of yourself. Take aspirin and drink lots of juice and rest. Otherwise, you will end up in the hospital or something."

"Can't I go to the doctor? Maybe I could get some pills to take to make me better."

"What doctor? What are you talking about? You have no doctor."

"But you and Sharon do. Maybe I could go to one of them."

"No, you can't. We both go to specialists. Mine is for arthritis and Sharon's is for her, well, you know, for her problem. They don't treat people like you, Paula. You're as healthy as a horse. They'd laugh at you for coming in and wasting their time."

"Wasting whose time?" Dad sat down at the kitchen table and started to unlace his work shoes.

"The doctor's time. She's not that sick; look at her, how big she is!"

Dad felt my forehead. "She feels pretty hot. Well, maybe we should call a doctor. Ronane's still over there. What time is it? Maybe he's still in his office."

Mother turned to look at the clock.

"It's after four. Close to four-thirty. I'm sure he's gone by this time. Besides, Ronane's a pediatrician. He'd probably love to get at someone as old and developed as Paula. It's just not a good idea."

My dad shrugged again.

"Well, we have to do something. She's been sick for a month, haven't you, Paula?"

I nodded, wiping my eyes and blowing thickly into a Kleenex. I looked dully from one to the other of my parents as they considered what to do with me.

"Isn't there a doctor across Greenfield, in those new brick offices?" Dad asked. " I thought you told me there were doctors in there."

"Who knows? Anyway, don't worry about it tonight. It's getting dark and it's cold and icy out there, and you need to stay in where it's warm after working outside all day. She'll be all right, won't you, Paula?"

I shivered and took another sip of the hot tea with honey and lemon that Mother had set before me on the table.

"Can I have some Throat Discs and that clear cough medicine? I ran out today. That stuff always makes me feel better."

Dad laughed.

"You mean that Terpin Hydrate Elixir? It should make you feel good. It's got codeine in it."

"What's codeine?"

"Never mind," Mother said. "It's just to quiet your cough, that's all. Why didn't you say something to Dad about going to the drug store before he took off his work boots? Now you want him to go back out in the cold, after he's been freezing all day like a popsicle. You can wait until tomorrow for that stuff, Paula. Dad will pick it up on his way home from work, won't you, Pops?"

A faint draft was blowing onto my bare feet from the side door. Shivering uncontrollably, I wrapped my arms tightly around my body, stood up, and shoved my chair under the table with my knee. I told my parents I was going to lie down, then went into the bathroom and warmed myself in front of the heating vent for 20 seconds before hurrying to bed where I lay shivering until I fell asleep.

The next morning I put on my warmest clothes: two thin flannel undershirts, navy woolen tights and an extra pair of knee socks, a divided slip, a white turtleneck, the forest green fur blend sweater and Pendleton wool black watch plaid coulottes Mother had given me for Christmas, and tall leather boots.

I was taking a chance to wear the coulottes on a day when I had civics class. Girls were not allowed to wear pants or shorts to school, and Miss Wasserfallen, the civics teacher, had an eagle's eye for finding the rule breakers whom she would lecture in a loud voice during her hall patrols before sending them to the office for a detention slip. But these were my heaviest winter clothes. At any other time I would have welcomed the chance to out fox the old girl, but my illness had made the coulottes a necessity. I was too sick to care whether I got caught; staying warm was everything.

I was at my locker after third period putting away my Latin book when I heard a jingle of keys behind me.

"You there. You, young lady. Please step away from your locker at once."

Without turning I recognized Wassy's authoritative voice.

I was right. There she stood, fleshy arms akimbo, hands on wide hips. Even in winter, she was wearing one of the bright pink, orange and red flower print dresses that turned her complexion florid, brought out the auburn highlights in her faded hair, and made me think once again of a plump summer squash.

Before she could speak I sneezed hard, twice, used two tissues to blow my nose, and coughed my barking cough.

"Oh, my, Paula. You sound so very sick!"

"I am, Miss Wasserfallen, and I know that you're going to send me to the office for wearing my coulottes, but I've got the chills and needed my warmest clothes today. I'm tempted to wear my winter jacket to class. Would you mind if I did?"

"Oh, my. You poor thing." Miss Wasserfallen held her hand gently to my forehead. "You are burning up with fever. Did your doctor give you permission to come to school?"

I pressed a Kleenex into my aching, burning eyes.

"I don't have a doctor. My mother said I was too old to go to the pediatrician, so my dad promised to go to the drug store tonight to get me cough drops."

"Cough drops! They won't do you a bit of good. You need antibiotics. Now then, come along with me. There's just enough time to get to the office before my next class."

I groaned inwardly. The witch! Miss Wasserfallen was exactly as everyone said, a tough old tank who mowed down even the most repentant rule breakers. I said nothing, but followed her down to the office, listening to her greet students along the way. She seemed to know everyone by name, but then she should; she was the only one who taught civics to the college prep students at Cooley High.

When we got to the office, Miss Wasserfallen asked, "Now, where do you live, dear?"

"I live on Rutherford and Six Mile. It's 17181 Rutherford," I replied. Was she going to send my detention slip to my parents?

"Please look under physicians in the Yellow Pages and help this young lady make an appointment to see a doctor in her neighborhood around Greenfield and Six Mile immediately," Miss Wasserfallen instructed the office secretary.

To me she said, "Now Paula, you are a fine young lady, always very polite and respectful, and an excellent student. I enjoy having you in my class. But sometimes one can be too conscientious. You must go to the doctor. The secretary will help arrange an appointment. Is there anyone at home who can come after you? No? Can we call your mother or father at work?"

Again I shook my head, no.

Miss Wasserfallen looked at me for a moment without speaking.

"If I didn't have a class now, I'd take you myself. But it can't be helped. I'm afraid you'll just have to go on your own."

She turned to the secretary.

"Please explain the circumstances to the doctor and see that they bill Paula's parents, or me, if necessary. Then call the transit authority and find out when this student's bus will be passing the school. It's too cold for her to be standing out waiting for it to come along. She can go out at the last minute to catch it."

Miss Wasserfallen rubbed her hand gently across my shoulders several times. The gesture warmed me.

"Now, dear, after you go to the doctor and get yourself some medicine, I want you to go home to bed and stay there until you are absolutely well. You're so sick that you also might be making your classmates ill. Don't worry about a thing, dear, except getting better. I'll see that one of your girlfriends calls you with homework assignments, but you're not to do a thing until you're really feeling up to it, do you understand?"

I raised my eyes and nodded. Miss Wasserfallen was smiling. She seemed less and less like the Nazi general we all had made her out to be.

"Thank you, Miss Wasserfallen." I hoped she thought the tears were from illness. I felt embarrassed, crying simply because she cared what happened to me.

The buses came like clock work: one down Hubbel to Six Mile, the next down Six Mile to the new brick building and the general practioner's office, just seven blocks from home.

"My nurse told me your teacher and a secretary at the high school helped you to find us. Is that correct?" the doctor asked. "Where is your mother? And your father, is he at work, too?

"Well, you have quite a friend in, what's her name, Miss Wasserfallen? Hmm. Miss Waterfall. Anyway, you must take very good care of yourself, Paula. Finish all of your medication, and call me if you think you need more. You have walking pneumonia. People die from that, you know."

I walked the seven blocks to Rutherford, then walked four more blocks beyond that to Smith's Drugs where the doctor had arranged for me to charge the perscription, before retracing my steps home. As I came in the side door and stepped into the kitchen, I paused for a moment as I took my medicine to consider the coffee rings on the counter top and the dirty dishes in the sink.

Then I hung up my coat, changed my clothes, and climbed into bed. As I settled under the cozy blankets and slippery quilts, I heard the Nancy Drew book and the paper dolls slide off and strike the floor.

Chapter 25

The Holy City

The telephone in the hallway of our home in Detroit, a thousand miles from Masaryktown, Florida, rang once, twice, three, then four times.

"Do you want me to get it?" I called into the night, across to my parents' bedroom.

"No, don't let her answer, Paul. You go." My mother's voice was hushed. "When phones ring at this hour, it's always bad news. Go, go answer it."

"Yes, operator, yes, go ahead. Hello? Yes? Oh? Oh. Geez!" Dad's voice grew louder, sharper as he spoke. "When? Where is he now? How's my mother? Good. Well, thank you for being there. Will someone stay with her until I come? I'll be there sometime tomorrow. You'll tell her? Good. Okay. Goodnight."

From where I lay I could see my father's hand resting on the receiver, long after he'd hung up the phone. "What's wrong, Dad? What happened?"

"Pappy--Grandpa--died tonight. In the kitchen. After supper. I'll fly down there tomorrow to take care of arrangements. You kids go back to sleep. I have to call Uncle John and Aunt Helen and Auntie Ann. Go on now, lay down and go to sleep."

The next morning as Mother got ready for work and we dressed for school, Dad called the airlines for flight information.

"How much more would it be for two?" he asked before hanging up.

"Is Mother going with you?" I asked.

"Mother doesn't want to come. She says she's afraid to fly, and that you should go. You come with me, Paula."

I hesitated.

"But I'll miss school."

"Just one day. Well, two. You can make up the work. It's for a funeral. They'll let you make it up."

Still, I hesitated.

"Where will we stay? In a motel?"

"Uh-uh. At Grandma's house."

"Will she be there with us?"

"Why, sure. Where else is she going to go? With Grandpa?"

I hurried to pack, then dressed in my black knit, longsleeved church dress with the black crocheted lace around the low V-neck. I put on nylons and black high heels, lipstick and eye makeup.

"Better keep an eye on her, Paul," Mother warned, giving me an appraising look. "Some Spic will come along when you aren't looking and kidnap her to Cuba."

Dad laughed.

"Don't worry, I won't let her out of my sight the whole trip," he promised.

That evening, I watched the tiny white moths flutter near the fluorescent ceiling lights in Grandma's kitchen with its shiny, pale grey walls as she sat in her cotton house dress and one of Grandpa's engulfing, dark wool coat sweaters.

She greeted her visitors in the warm room: Placko, Hlavac, Funtik, Nemec, Vohun, one-eyed Ventura, Slavs who had grown old farming in the tiny Czech settlement. She rocked back and forth in her straight-back chair, and in cracked words and broken sentences told and retold the story of my grandfather's death.

"Pavel was sitting there, that's right, right there, at the table. He finished his supper, and was sitting, resting, you know, and not saying much. Well, he was tired. He'd worked all day long, and it was late. Then he just stood up, and I thought he was going to bed. But he didn't go to his room. He went to that door." Grandma nodded toward the heavy door that led to the parlor. "And he went in, put on a light by the organ, and began to play."

It was at this point that her story would be interrupted by shoulder-shaking sobs.

"He hadn't...he hadn't played the organ in five, ten years. But he went in, sat down, and started singing and playing 'The Holy City'. It was his favorite hymn. Paula, Paula, my granddaughter, come here to Grandma, Paula, you play it for them so that they'll know. And sing, sing for Grandma."

I entered the cold, dark parlor, groped for the light, seated myself on the high, creaky bench, looked around for Grandpa's ghost, then pulled out the stops and, pumping the bellows with my feet, began to play and sing Grandpa's favorite song. I could hear Grandma's cries wrack the air as I finished the music, and she, her story:

"Then Pavel came back into the kitchen," my grandmother explained. "He shut the door so that the cold from the parlor wouldn't come in, sat down in his chair, put his hand over his heart like this, lay his head down on the table... and just went to sleep."

The visitors wept, rubbed Grandma's shoulders, cupped her trembling hands, said a word of prayer or read from the Slovak Bible opened on the faded oil cloth, and went out into the night. It was cold, and the farmhouse had no central heat. I shivered near Grandma's small electric heater. Finally, she led the way from the kitchen into the front bedroom where Dad had put our suitcase.

"Paula, you go on, get dressed for bed. Do you have a warm nightgown to wear? If not, I have some for you. Now go, get washed up, it's late. When you're done, come kiss Grandma goodnight."

When I returned to the bedroom in my flannel gown, warm socks, and an old robe from behind the bathroom door that went twice around me, Grandma was laying down-filled quilts that she and Grandpa had made across the bed.

Dad was lifting things out of his case to get to his pajamas.

"Where am I sleeping tonight, Grandma?" I asked.

"In here. It's cold, but these nice quilts Grandpa made will keep you warm."

"Where is Dad sleeping?"

My father was looking for his pajamas in the suitcase.

"That's too many, Ma," he said, turning to look at the bed.

"We'll be too hot."

Grandma looked from me to him, then questioned him sharply in Czech.

Dad answered in his mother's language.

"No," she said. "It's not right."

He pulled a quilt off the bed, grabbed a pillow, and went into the parlor.

Grandma look hard into my face.

"He won't be sleeping with you any more," she said. And she tucked the covers in around me.

Chapter 26

Scenes

I rushed to the rear of the apartment and stood there with my hands clasped behind me, rocking on my heels and grinning. As I held open the back door, he brushed past me and walked into the kitchen. He eyed the pile of dirty baking utensils and the bowl, clotted with the first recipe of double laundry starch that I had ever mixed.

"What the hell have you been doing all day?"

I quailed for an instant at his scowl, then brightened.

"Well, there's this," I said, reaching for the fresh blueberry pie--his favorite--that had been cooling on top of the refrigerator.

"And then there are these." He followed me to the bedroom where I stood, proudly displaying the two newly ironed shirts.

"I spent an hour on each of these."

He took one of them from me and carried it to the window, where he inspected it closely in the light.

"This one has a wrinkle on the pocket. Give me the other. And look at this." He thrust the second shirt in front of me and pointed to a tiny crease on the left shoulder. "What do you take me for, some kind of bum? I can't be seen in public wearing something that looks like this."

He yanked the shirts off their hangers, balled them tightly together, then threw them into the clothes hamper.

He was about to turn and walk out of the bedroom, but

instead he moved toward the neatly made bed, grabbed the covers, and pulled them back. Then he took something from his pocket, stepped back and threw it. The quarter landed with a dull thud in the center of the mattress.

"You can't even make a bed right," he yelled, tearing off the sheet. "Now put it on again, and this time, pull it taut. A bed isn't made correctly unless a quarter can bounce on it!"

He threw the sheet at me.

"I always said you were only good for one thing."

There was a river at the bottom of our street, and a big park with lawns smooth as handkerchiefs and paths as hard and brown as drum heads made of skin. I loved to take the neighbor's Alaskan malamute running in the park, and one evening as I did so, a storm came up. Since there was no lightning, I ran on, but by the time I got home, I was drenched and cold. He was at the back door, waiting, I thought, with a towel. But his clenched hands were empty.

"Where the hell were you? Didn't you know I'd be worried sick about you, you dummy? Now, tell me where you were and who you were with!"

I tried to walk past him to the bathroom for a towel, but he blocked my way. When I wedged myself between him and the wall, he suddenly grabbed me around the shoulders and sent me reeling against the kitchen cupboards. Then he grabbed my arm and twisted it and twisted it until I cried out in pain.

"Well, you deserve to be punished, after causing me all that worry! Next time, it will be much worse!"

At the hospital, he stayed near the X-ray technician.

Later, he stood facing me from behind the nurses as they asked again and again how I had hurt my arm. And each time, I told the story he and I had carefully rehearsed. I was faithful to the smallest detail.

On the way home, it was as if he could read my mind.

"Don't think for a minute that I'm sorry for what happened tonight," he said as he drove down the deserted road. "You got just what you deserved for being out when you belong at home with me. And don't even think about running away. I know your Social Security number and I have friends in the police. I'll keep looking until I find you, and when I do, I'll kill you--then I'll turn the gun on myself."

Chapter 27

In Another Country

My husband told me he was leaving the marriage one December. It was Christmas week, and I was lying in a hospital bed one day after surgery. I made no reply. I couldn't; I had just had a tonsilectomy.

The marriage ended two weeks later on my daughter's fourth birthday. Ivan helped his dad pack a suitcase, and he was gone. Three days later, Ivan was covered with chicken pox. Three months later, I was denied tenure at Adrian College, a small Christian school in southeastern Michigan to which I had commuted eighty miles daily during six school years to teach English and journalism in a department where everyone else was tenured--and male.

While I could return to Adrian to teach for another year, it was time to start looking for other employment. My mother would call periodically and blame me that the marriage was over, that Ivan and Claire would be latchkey kids in a broken home:

"Hello, Paula, this is Mother. How are you, honey? Do you need anything? Can Dad and I help?"

"Thanks for offering, Mother, but we really don't need anything right now. We'll be okay. The kids are great."

"Poor little kids! My goodness! They're like a couple of little orphans. No father, and a mother who goes off and leaves them all the time. "

"You make it sound like a crime that I have to work, Mother. We've got to eat, to live. In order to do that, I have to work."

"Work, my eye! If you hadn't wrecked your marriage and let such a good guy go, you'd never have to work. But no; you go off and dessert your children and a husband who kept the house and the children so nice and neat and clean, and what do you have left? Nothing! Well, it serves you right. You've dug your hole, now lay in it."

But Jeannette Leahy, my dear secretary, was forever in support of me, of my ability to mother, to teach. It was Jeannette who began slipping want ads from the Chronicle of Higher Education, the Detroit Free Press, and the Toledo Blade into my mailbox. It was Jeannette who typed my resume and cover letters and helped me to arrange job interviews because I was too emotionally paralyzed to function. And it was Jeannette who supported my decision to turn down job offers in Michigan and Ohio and head south to Kentucky, a place where, because of its physical beauty, I'd always dreamed of living.

And so, still emotionally and physically bereft from an unhappy marriage of more than ten years, torn from the house in Toledo where I had lived for more than eight years that my children remembered as "home," uprooted from my beloved yard where the trees and flowers at last had bloomed in succession, we moved to Bowling Green so that I could teach at Western Kentucky University.

Today, I love Bowling Green, which will remain forever in my heart as my first real home, and her people, my people. But in those days, I hated the town and its smallness, and what I construed as a lack of things to do because I was too angry and depressed to do them. At first I couldn't communicate with these Southerners who made single-syllable words into two, and two syllable words into one--never mind that they couldn't understand my Michigan accent. Their warmth, their friendliness, was as foreign to my suspicious Yankee mind as was their food. I would look in bewilderment at the corn cakes stacked on plates of barbecue and greens and wonder why Southerners ate pancakes without syrup for lunch. I was in another country.

During those early months in Bowling Green I felt truly in pain, alienated, alone, without friends save for my small son and daughter. It was Ivan who finally helped to change that. One day as we were waiting to turn at the light at Twelfth and Chestnut streets to go to the university, Ivan looked at the big church on the corner.

"Mama, can we go there on Sunday?" he asked, nodding toward the First Baptist Church building.

"There, Ivan?" The grey walls looked cold, austere. "Why do you want to go there?"

"I like the way the church looks outside, and I want to see it from the inside. I want to see the stained glass windows. And the tower."

"Do you mean the dome? I guess that would be pretty neat to see. And the windows look like they're pale pink and green. They're unusual. I guess we could go, just once."

I didn't want to go to First Baptist or to any other church. Not only was the thought of smiling and shaking the hands of strangers unbearable to me, but so was the thought of worshipping a God who had clearly deserted me. I never wanted to enter a church again, but I couldn't deny my son that privilege, and so, on Sunday, we went.

Ivan and Claire were whisked away to their appropriate Sunday School classes. I was directed across the parking lot to a white frame building that housed the Cambodian and the Singles Sunday schools, up a narrow, creaking staircase, and into a classroom. It belonged to Mary Dillingham, my daughter's first grade teacher.

Mary's blue dress matched her eyes, and her sterling jewelry, her prematurely silver hair. She was stunning; and as she smiled and made room for me in the circle of 10 women and one man, I was taken by her warmth. I could see that we all were. Drawn to Mary Dillingham's class by the common bond of loss through divorce or death, we went each week, not so much to hear Baptist dogma, but for emotional support to mend our broken spirits. Mary was our healer.

"What is the very first commandment?" she asked one Sunday as she looked around the group and smiled.

"'Love thy neighbor as thy self,'" a number of us chorused.

"That's the first verse. But what is the very first commandment?" she asked again.

We looked at each other, puzzled, curious.

"Is it 'Love thy neighbor?'" our teacher asked.

I, for one, nodded yes.

"I'm not so sure," she said gently. "To me, the first commandment comes in the second half of the verse--'as thyself.' Do you see? You have to love yourself before you can love your neighbor--or anyone. If you haven't learned how to love yourself, how can you possibly know how to love another?"

Had someone dropped a feather, each of us would have heard it touch the earth.

She went on in her gentle voice:

"We're taught all our lives to live for others, to care for others, to give to others, that to think of ourselves and our own needs is wrong, is selfish. But if we don't take care of our own needs, who will? Nobody. Yet we keep on giving, neglecting what we want, and little by little, we become angry and resentful.

"Then one day, when there's nothing of us left because we've given it all away, the frustration becomes too much and our marriages end. Or the anger spills over, and we die. That's why God gave that commandment first--it's both the most important and most difficult thing to do--to learn to love ourselves, just as we are."

By that time each of us was crying or speechless or nodding at the truth in Mary's words. Most of us had been brought up on that commandment, and had devoted our lives entirely to others--wasn't that what Christianity was all about? No. And it was right there, all the time, in the very first verse.

" Now it is time to stop giving all of ourselves to others," Mary said. "It is time to stop feeling guilty. It is time for each of us to start caring for ourselves."

Before we left the Sunday School class Mary asked each of us to describe something loving and special we would do for ourselves that day that wouldn't cost anything. One woman loved hats; she would spend the afternoon at the mall trying them on. Another planned to rake her yard and hang Indian corn on her front door in celebration of autumn, the season of her birth. Still another loved to walk; she would go hiking at Mammoth Cave.

That afternoon I waved Ivan and Claire out the back door to play with their friends in the yard, set a kettle of water to boil on the stove, and stacked kindling and logs in the fireplace of our apartment.

Later, as I stretched out on the couch in the warmth of the blaze, I said a prayer of thanks for Mary Dillingham's wisdom and for the beginning of my awakening, my release. Then I slowly poured hot Earl Grey tea into my favorite china tea cup; it had been packed away for months.

Chapter 28

Christmas Reunion

The days hurtled into years, years of anger, years of hatred, years of resentment. I saw my sister once in all of those years, at a family reunion one Christmas when my parents were living in Southgate, Michigan.

I saw dear aunts and uncles whom I had not seen for a long time, even though I was living only two or three hours away from most of them. My marriage was like my childhood: reclusive, suspicion-filled, untrusting. I saw few people, had few friends. My relatives were not numbered among them.

"Why don't you ever go to see your aunts and uncles?" my mother would sometimes ask. "You drive. Just get in the car and go without that husband of yours."

"No, I don't really like to go visiting alone, and he says that Sundays are his only day to rest, so we just don't do much with other people."

"I'll bet you see his family."

"Well, we do, but not that often. Sometimes he goes over there alone."

"Well, Paula, you should stop feeling sorry for yourself. Remember what the Old Testament says: 'Ye shall leave your parents and cleave to your husband and your husband's people.'"

The Christmas reunion was happy in all ways but one: my sister, her husband and her sons were there. I couldn't bring myself to look at her boys; they looked too much like Sharon. Was I afraid that I would resent them, too?

I could say the estrangement had occured because my sister had married a soldier in the army during the Vietnam War years, and our politics clashed. Young as I was, I believed that war was wrong, and suddenly I had a brother-in-law who fought in one.

But no, that was just an excuse hiding the deep resentment I felt toward Sharon because of our mother's special treatment of her as a somewhat feeble minded invalid who was physically too weak to help much with housework and mentally and physically unable to withstand punishment of any sort.

Ivan was only two at the Christmas reunion. There was a present for him under the tree.

"Ivan, come here, sweetheart, see what Grandma has for you," my mother called to him.

She handed him a gailey wrapped package.

"This is for you, sweetie. Here, give Grandma a kiss."

She gave Ivan a squeeze and a kiss on the cheek, and then let him go to open his present. My aunts and uncles, none of whom had granchildren of their own, smiled and watched.

 Suddenly two slightly larger hands--my nephew's--appeared out of nowhere, grabbed the present from Ivan, tore off the paper, and tossed the gift back at him. Ivan ran to show me: it was a bright red and brown stuffed Curious George. Ivan looked at George, ran to hug my mother again, then ran to me to show me the gift that, then and there, became the pal which he carried day and night for years, always tucked under his left arm.

But instead of being delighted over Ivan's pleasure with his new baby, Mother focused on what had happened after she handed Ivan his present.

"He didn't even get to open his own gift," she muttered to me as we carried plates of pickles, olives, radishes, celery and carrot sticks to the dining room. "Sharon's kids are brats! They've only been here two days and they're driving us crazy. They yell and throw pillows at each other, and one of them, the younger one--you know, the one who grabbed Ivan's present and tore it open--was running down the hallway yesterday and bumped right into your father! It makes me so damn mad! Dad could have been hurt, and then what? So he made them put on their jackets and hats and he locked them outside for an hour. They're really army brats! They're devils!"

"Well, Mother, they're just kids with a lot of energy to burn. Just concentrate on how much Ivan loves his Curious George, and how much we appreciate the gift."

"Kids, my foot. They're brats, and that's all there is to it. We should never have invited Sharon and Steve to stay here."

I said nothing, but I silently agreed, adding the incident to the huge stockpile of injustices I felt my sister had done to me over the years. Of course they were brats. After all, they were my sister's children; what else could they be?

Chapter 29

At the Winn-Dixie

When I moved to Bowling Green in a state of perpetual depression, I felt as I had 10 years earlier when, as a graduate student at the University of Toledo where I studied psychoanalysis and literature, I had suffered a nervous breakdown and been hospitalized so that I would not kill myself. Try as I might, I couldn't think clearly. I would force myself to focus on the simplest of tasks, then give up in the middle of them. I recall one day being unable to remember how to peel a cucumber.

Now it amazes me that I was able to get up each morning, see Ivan, then 8, and Claire, then 6, off to school each day on the bus, shower, dress and drive to the university to teach four journalism classes. I must have done it by rote and through luck. I had been a professional journalist, had taught some of the material at Adrian College in Michigan. The students seemed to be learning; they even seemed to like me. But it boggled my mind that they could, for I was a hypocrite, a sham who longed not to be talking with them in my office, but curled up alone at home, in bed.

And what was home to us now? We'd left a two story house and moved into a two-bedroom apartment. Each of us had brought our clothes, a bed and a chest of drawers, along with a couch, table and lamp for the living room and kitchen utensils and linens. We'd left our most familiar and beloved possessions--the toys, the books, the pictures, the piano, the antiques--in storage in Toledo, Ohio. We had brought only what we absolutely needed, what would fit in the small U-Haul truck, the one we could afford to rent.

I felt so physically and emotionally bereft that I would go to that apartment when I was done teaching my morning classes and sleep for hours, or sit, staring into space, with but a single thought on my mind: to kill myself.

I had stopped eating much of anything the year of the divorce. Grocery shopping and cooking became insurmountable tasks. It was Ivan who would inform me, encourage me, goad me to buy food so that he and Claire would have something to eat.

The thought of my hungry children would somehow propel me to action, even as I was berating myself for being so unloving, inconsiderate, incompetent, just the kind of mother my former husband had often accused me of being.

We would drive, or often walk, the three of us, across the rutted, weedy fields past Bowling Green High to the Wynn-Dixie on Scottsville Road, where Ivan would help Claire climb into a grocery cart and place my hands on the handles as I stared hopelessly, vacantly ahead. Then he would scoot up and under, and together, we would begin pushing the cart.

"Did you bring the list?" he would ask.

"List?" I'd look down at him, puzzled. "What list?"

"You know, Mama, the grocery list. Remember? Claire and I figured out what we needed and then I wrote it all down so you wouldn't have to. Don't you remember? You were sitting in the kitchen watching us."

But no, I couldn't remember. I would start pushing the cart vacantly up one aisle and down another, through the produce department, past the canned soups and spaghetti, the bread, the milk, the lunchmeat. Had Ivan not tossed items in the cart, each time glancing at me cautiously to see if I was mad, or crying, it would have remained empty as we got to the checkout lanes.

One blustery afternoon in early spring we drove to the Winn-Dixie. Ivan was in front with me, holding his shopping list.

"We only need a few things, Mama," he said. "Then we can come right home so that you can go back to bed."

I nodded absently. Ivan got the cart, and once again, we walked the aisles while Claire rode.

"Here's the macaroni and cheese, Mama. We'll have that with hotdogs for dinner, o.k.?"

I took the package from him, looked at it, then made him put it back.

"I can't let you kids eat that stuff, Ivan. It's full of salt. It would taste terrible. We'll find something else."

Each time he and his little sister chose something--chicken noodle soup and crackers, a jar of spaghetti sauce--I would say "no." At the end of our shopping trip there was only one thing in the basket--a gallon jug of milk.

"Mama, aren't we going to buy anyting else? There's no food for supper." Ivan looked worried.

"Can't I have a box of Honey Nut Cheerios? Ivan put them on the list," Claire said.

"No. No sugar foods. No junk. That's all we ever eat. Come on. Let's go. There's food at home." I felt angry and tired. I needed to lie down.

Back at the apartment, Ivan put the milk away, then reported back to me.

"We have three pieces of bread and one slice of cheese. That's all. And the milk."

I was already half asleep on the couch. My head hurt, and I felt disoriented.

"Uh-huh. Don't worry about it. I won't let you kids go hungry. Just let me sleep a little while and then we'll go to the store."

I felt two small hands tuck a blanket in around me, and I slept. When I awoke later, it was dark. I could hear the soft whispers of my children in the kitchen. I could smell hotdogs cooking. I got up slowly and went in to sit at the kitchen table.

"Oh, hi, Mama, are you feeling better?" Claire put her small arms around me and gave me a kiss.

"How about some supper, Mama? I'm cooking hotdogs with bread and Franco American spaghetti." Ivan stood back from the stove and proudly displayed the steaming pots.

"Where did that come from, Ivan? Where did you get the food?"

"After you laid down I thought you'd probably sleep for a long time, like you usually do, and Claire and I were hungry, so I took five dollars from your purse and rode to Wynn-Dixie on my bike. I only bought what I could carry, and I have your change right here. I hope you're not mad that I did that."

Hot tears stung my eyes. I stretched out my arms and held my son and my daughter tightly.

"Thank you for taking such good care of us, Sweetie," I said.

"I don't know what's wrong with me, why I'm always so tired, why I don't want to eat. But I need to take better care of you kids."

Ivan got three plates from the cupboard and started dishing out the food.

"Just get better, Mama. And don't worry about anything. I'll take care of you and Claire. I'm the man in the family now, with Daddy gone."

A sudden fury raged within me. I put Claire aside and was across the kitchen in two strides, my hands on Ivan's shoulders, gripping him so tightly he looked frightened.

"You are not the man in the family. There is no man in this family anymore. There's only one adult here, and that's me," I said, amazed at my sudden energy, sparked by this current of hot anger that surged up, out of nowhere. "You are the boy in the family and Claire is the girl in the family, and that's how I want it to stay! You are children--not little adults. I don't want you to worry or work. I want you to laugh and to play, to have friends. Please! Have the childhood that I ... that I ...

The hot tears spilled down my cheeks. I could not finish the sentence.

Something had happened. I had broken through.

Then we sat down, gave thanks, and ate.

Chapter 30

Watch

At midnight, the only light in the room came from the numbers of the digital clock on the nightstand. It shone on the untouched glasses of burgundy that were beginning to sour, and on the jumble of dirty sheets.

My boyfriend of two years bumped up the dark stairway, then stumbled against the bedroom door. It flew open, hitting the wall.

"Who's there? Who is it?"

He crossed the room to the bed. As he gropped for the slender neck of the nightable lamp with the cupids on the shade, his hand hit one of the glasses. Wine spilled everywhere.

"What's wrong? Are you drunk? What happened?"

I was sitting up, looking into his face. He did not answer, but drew something from the pocket of his coat. It was a watch of dull gold. The band was a string of hearts. He pulled it over his fingers, stretching the band.

"Oh. It's so beauti--." I stopped myself as I stared at the watch. "Wait a minute. Isn't that hers? Isn't that her watch?"

"That's right. I gave it to her for our anniversary. She said she wouldn't need it anymore. That it was broken and couldn't be fixed."

He pulled the watch up higher on his white knuckles where they were making a fist.

"But maybe it can be fixed," I said, reaching for the watch.

"No. Don't. Don't touch it."

He jerked the watch around until I could see the face. The crystal was crushed. The hands were stopped at three o'clock. I sucked in my breath.

"But why? Why would the bitch destroy something so beautiful? Did she really hate you that much?"

He did not reply at first, but stood staring at the watch. Then he spread the fingers of his broad hand wide, stretching the band taut.

"She said she was awake when they did it. She said just before they took it that she handed the watch to a nurse and had her step on it. She said she told them that the watch would be the only thing from me that she would have left and that she would be giving it back."

He and I looked at the watch. When the band snapped, hearts went everywhere. Suddenly he bent down, picked up the watch, and threw it as hard as he could at the wall. A piece of pink paint and plaster hit the floor.

He turned and stared at me, but it appeared that he did not see me.

"The bitch," he said through clenched teeth.

"Dad? Daddy? What are you doing up there? Is Paula with you?"

His son's voice stirred him. He went to the head of the stairs.

"Don't come up! Stay downstairs. Didn't I tell you before? Didn't I say don't come up this time for any reason? Didn't I? Answer me! Didn't I?"

The boy made some reply.

"Don't argue! Go back and lie down in the family room. Now!"

When he re-entered the bedroom he closed the door carefully, pressing a warped corner shut with the flat of his hand. Then he crossed the room to the bed. He stood above me, staring down at me, unbuckling his belt.

"What are you doing? Are you going to lay down? Here. Come lay down beside me."

I sat up, knelt on the bed, and fixed two pillows for him.

"There!" I said, fluffing the pillows. "What you need is a good night's..."

Suddenly he grabbed my long hair by the roots and yanked my head around. His penis was erect, purple, as he shoved it into my mouth. I struggled against him, gasping and gagging. The harder I fought, the deeper his fingers wound in my hair, pulling it.

He loosened his hold on me abruptly. But before I could slide away from him, he shoved me down on the mattress and pressed his left hand between my breasts. With his right hand, he worked his pants and underwear down around his ankles.

"You better not scream, bitch, don't scream."

I turned my head to one side, took a deep breath, and screamed. He grabbed a pillow and held it, hard, over my face with his left hand. He pinned me down with the weight of his upper body. I struggled for air as he pushed up my nightgown, tore off my panties, and pushed my thighs apart. He missed twice before he penetrated. His size and the power of his thrusts made me cry out.

"The bitch, the bitch, the bitch, the bitch, the bitch, the bitch, the bitch. Bitch! Bitch! Bitch!"

Chapter 31

Healing Angels

There are those who have been sexually, physically and emotionally abused who discharge their rage through violence toward others; they are the thieves, the drug dealers, the rapists, the murderers who kill for a nickel or for the hell of it.

Then there are the rest of us: we take that same rage and direct the violence at ourselves. Many of us have been raised on religious beliefs. We agree that murder is wrong, is horrifying; for us, it is beyond imagination to kill someone. Yet we see nothing immoral about murdering ourselves, because for most of our lives we have been taught that we are worthless, and have grown to believe it.

But do we really want to die?

Often I did want to die; but sometimes I didn't. And I told this to Mary Elizabeth Hickman through tearful sobs one day as I sat in her Nashville office. It was the fifth or sixth time in three weeks that I had driven the 65 miles to see the therapist. Between appointments, she had also kept track of me through daily long distance calls she made at her own expense. She wanted to make sure that I was still alive.

"Why do you think you want to kill yourself?" she asked me gently one day in her office.

"I don't know. I don't know." The Kleenex in my hands was a tangled shred. Mary Elizabeth placed a box of tissues beside me, then waited. "Sometimes I don't want to die. But at other times, I feel so victimized by suicide--it seems like the only answer to all of these damned problems."

Suddenly she sat forward. "Paula, what did you just say--about victimization--I mean?"

I thought for a minute. "Well, sometimes, when things are going smoothly, I might think of suicide and, intellectually, it seems like a such a strange idea; it's almost foreign to me--as if that impulse belongs to somebody else. But then something happens, and there I am again, back in the pit of despair with that beast over me, reaching, clawing at me.

"Take last week, for example. Ivan, Claire and I were doing okay at the beginning. The weather was so beautiful that we took a couple of long walks and got lots of sleep. I was all caught up in my classes and with other work at my office. But then Claire came home with the flu. Ivan got it next, and it went into an ear infection. I was up late some nights taking care of both of them. I fell behind in grading papers. I had to run around to doctors' offices and the grade school to pick up the kids' books and assignments when I was supposed to be at the university holding office hours. I tend to worry about my job a lot. I guess when you lose one, you live in fear of the next.

"Then I got sick, and then I got depressed. Or maybe I got stressed out and angry and then became depressed, and then I got sick. Who knows? The point is that I can remember so clearly two weeks ago not feeling suicidal, and now all I can think of is to kill myself. I can't think clearly, I can't breathe, I can hardly move my arms and legs, they feel so heavy. I hate to feel this way. But I don't know how not to, and try as I might, I can't seem to pull myself out of it. Well meaning friends used to tell me to just pull myself up by my bootstraps. Anyone who says that has no idea what depression is really like."

Mary Elizabeth waited while I dried my eyes and blew my nose. I shrugged. "I just feel so hopeless--and helpless."

Once again, she leaned toward me. Her tone was even:

"Paula, I just know that I can help you, because you want to be helped, but I can't do it alone. I want you to do something for me."

I looked up at her surprised, curious. While I could rarely accept help from others, I was always willing to give it. What could I do for my therapist?

"Paula--" she hesitated. "I know you don't want to take any medication. You told me during your first visit that a psychiatrist in Toledo had once prescribed anit-depressants, but that the side effects were so bad, you took yourself off.

"But, Paula--" she stopped again as if in frustration that the right words, the ones that would convince me to cooperate, might not come. "I discussed your case with a friend--a colleague--this week because I felt he could help you. Now I'm convinced. Anyone who talks about being victimized by suicide is not suicidal."

I was beginning to feel somehow angry and betrayed that Mary Elizabeth had discussed my case without my permission. But it was as if she had read my thoughts:

"I hope you don't feel that I've gone behind your back; please believe that I would never betray a client's trust. This friend is Kirby Pate--Dr. J. Kirby Pate--a psychiatrist. He's young, and he was a Fellow in psychiatry at Vanderbilt Medical School, so he's extremely bright. And he's also very nice. I think you'd like him. He only wants to visit with you for about 30 minutes, and he's willing to see you any time that it would be convenient for you, even on a Saturday. His office is only a few blocks from here. And Paula," she added gently, "you won't get lost. I promise."

What was it that made me agree to meet with Dr. Pate the following Saturday afternoon? Was it those long distance calls that Mary Elizabeth made, simply because she cared what happened to me? Or, was it that she believed that I didn't really want to kill myself?

Dr. Pate's greeting was warm and quiet. He assured me that he would not keep me long, asked me to sit down, handed me a list of foods, and asked if I tended to crave any of them. I read him my choices, about half the list:

"Chocolate, buttermilk, aged cheeses such as blue and sharp cheddar, pickles and olives, preserved meats including hard salami, raisins, and very ripe bananas. How am I doing?"

Dr. Pate smiled. "Unfortunately, you're doing very well. Numerous studies indicate that these are among the foods that people who suffer from clinical depression often crave.

"Let me ask you this: do you tend to be more depressed at certain times of the year than others? And, what about bedtime?

"If you had no family or work or social responsibilities at night, when would you prefer to go to sleep?"

I told him I often suffered the greatest depression around Labor Day, and through the winter months. It seemed to subside with the time change in the spring. I also said that I would love to go to bed around 8 p.m. and wake up at 3:30 or 4 a.m. I had done it a few times, and had always awakened feeling alert and alive.

I actually smiled at the thought. "It's wonderful. I love sunset and sunrise, and on those days, I was able to be outside for both."

The psychiatrist explained that depressed people seem to require greater amounts of ultraviolet light than do the nondepressed. He said it was only logical that depression increases as the daylight hours decrease in the fall and winter months.

"We can also blame some of the depression on Thomas Edison."

"Edison?"

"That's right. There was far less incidence of depression reported in the nineteenth century and earlier than there is now," he said. "People went to bed at sundown and got up at sunrise. In other words, they were getting the optimum levels of natural light, and probably living by their internal clocks. But when Tom Edison came along with his light bulb, folks just stayed up later. They got fewer ultraviolet rays at the same time that they unwittingly tampered with their internal clocks. And we've been doing it ever since, much to the detriment of depressed people.

"Your responses to my questions, coupled with the consultation about you that I had with Mrs. Hickman a day or two ago lead me to believe very strongly that you have a chemical imbalance that is highly treatable with the right medication.

"Mrs. Hickman also explained to me that you take pride in being self-reliant and would prefer not to use medication, especially since you had a bad experience with anti-depressants in the past. Yet we both feel certain that with the proper dosage of the anti-depressant that's just right for your condition, within just a few weeks, you'd start to feel like an entirely different person."

Just then, a new wave of despair washed over me, and I began to cry.

"Something I just said upset you," Dr. Pate said quietly. "Can you tell me why you're crying?"

I shrugged. "I don't like to depend on things outside of myself, like medication. And that other medicine made me feel dried out all the time, and really uncomfortable. And I don't really have the money or the time to spend both with you and Mary Elizabeth."

"I'm not interested in keeping patients in therapy for years and years. I just want them to get well. I think your case involves a treatable imbalance that would respond quickly and well to medication. I feel certain that you would feel as if you had been reborn and were a brand new human being who could feel happiness and hope much of the time. I can almost guarantee it. Then the counseling that Mrs. Hickman is giving you will really be meaningful and helpful."

He paused and thought for a moment.

"I'll tell you what," he said. "Since you plan to meet regularly with Mrs. Hickman, she can advise me of your progress if you agree to go on medication. But you have to give the medicine at least six weeks to really take effect, and you have to notify me by phone immediately if there are any problems. I'll need to see you in seven to eight weeks. And one other thing--you have to give me your word that you won't use the Norpramin I'm going to prescribe to commit suicide."

It was that last stipulation that made me agree to try the drug. Somebody who could be that straight with me, that trusting, deserved my cooperation--but only for eight weeks.

Two months later, I was, in some ways, another person. While suicide remained a very clear option, I would consider killing myself, say, only three times a day instead of the usual five. The highs and lows began to level off. I was smiling, and even laughing more; I could breathe; the heaviness in my chest had dissipated; I had more energy to do things--including to very slowly begin taking a harder look at myself and how I had developed a suicidal personality.

I met with Mary Elizabeth once or twice a week for nearly two years. During the first three or four months of counseling, I did little more than cry. But not once did my therapist tell me that I had nothing to cry about, as my mother often had:

"Don't you mouth off to me! Don't you get angry at your parents!" My mother would shout as she drew back her hand and hit me across the face. "God punishes bad people, and angry people are the worst. With all your black marks, you'll burn in Hell for eternity, Paula! Just keep your feelings to yourself. "

Instead, Mary Elizabeth encouraged me to cry as often as I needed to get out all of the anger, the rage that I had stuffed deep inside me . She reminded me over and over that we are entitled to our feelings. She spent months demonstrating to me that because of the way we are treated in close relationships, children from emotionally, physically or sexually abusive homes are taught self-hatred rather than self-love.

"Maybe your parents were abused, but they won't say, because you've asked them, isn't that right? What you're trying to do, Paula, is break that cycle of abuse. Suicide is a choice that some people make. But there are other choices. There are also ways to break the cycle. I want to show you those other ways."

A first step was exercise, a formidable assignment for a depressed person, but one that I needed to cultivate because hard physical activity releases a chemical in the brain that eases depression. Mary Elizabeth wisely left the ways--and the amounts--up to me. She never chastized me for doing too little. I described to her days when I would get dressed to go out for a walk and end up sitting on the couch in despair.

But there were other days, days when I did get out the door and down the road, walking, sometimes running with dogs in the neighborhood around the cornfields behind our apartment, past the fields blue with chicory and pink and purple with aster where gold finches rode the wild grasses and blue jays stole sunflower seed, days that made me feel alive and well. It was my sheer love of nature and the beauty of natural light rather than the exercise itself that the therapist emphasized, and her wise approach encouraged me to turn more and more to nature--and exercise--for healing.

Another of the therapist's early goals was to help me build self-esteem. I had to do sensual things for myself and think about how good they made me feel.

"But I just don't have the money," I protested.

"The things I'm talking about won't cost anything, or very little. The point is to start doing loving things for yourself that you can take pleasure in. Put clean sheets on your bed and lie there and think about how good they feel next to your skin. Take a long, lingering bubblebath, and when you do, really enjoy the warmth of the water and the pretty bubbles. Don't do anything but lie there and think about how good you're feeling, how relaxed."

Mary Elizabeth opened our next counseling session by asking about my sensory experiences.

"One night I made myself a cup of Earl Grey tea, and really thought about how good it tasted."

The therapist smiled and nodded for me to go on.

"And then another night, after Ivan and Claire were asleep, I was piling more logs on the fire and I got some pine resin on my hands. It smelled so good that I left it on for awhile, so that I could keep enjoying it.

"And then, just last evening, I was in the doorway of my apartment doing what I always do when I'm at home. I was watching the sun set over the cornfields. The sky was streaked with lavender and peach, and the sun flamed orange as it disappeared, and everything was so still. I suddenly realized how much that experience means to me at the close of a day--" a sob caught in my throat--"and that... and that... I really don't want to miss a single sunset."

The therapist also gave me a list of some twenty statements. I was to read two or three of those aloud several times a day while looking at myself in a mirror until I could really feel the words and believe in them. I recall taking the list into the bathroom with me while I washed up for bed. I kept picking up the paper, then putting it down again. Finally, I took a deep breath. It was hard for me to raise my eyes and really look at myself in the mirror.

"I am a..." I lowered my eyes and took a deep breath. Then I tried again:

"I am a worthwhile..." a sob caught in my throat.

"I am a worthwhile--a worthwhile--person."

Chapter 32

My Sister, Sharon

It was Wednesday, February 14, Valentine's Day, and I called my sister, Sharon, who lives ten hours away by car in Alabama. Not an unusual occurrence for one sister to call another. But highly irregular for us. We had not spoken in more than 10 years.

There would be an occasional exchange of Christmas cards, a rare birthday card during that decade, sometimes photos of Sharon's sons, whom I'd met only once during the Christmas reunion at our parents' house in Southgate. I would look at the photographs and feel nothing, nothing at all, try as I might to make some emotional connection with those boys who grew into men in the envelopes.

According to our mother, my sister's future had been bleak; she had often said it would take a minor miracle for Sharon to find gainful employment. And marriage was clearly out of the question; no man, Mother reminded Sharon frequently, wants to marry damaged goods.

After several unsuccessful attempts at education following high school, Sharon went to work as a secretary. One day she went shopping in downtown Detroit, bought herself several new outfits, beautiful clothes and shoes at J.L. Hudson when it was still a fine department store on Woodward Avenue, and told me that she had arranged to take a trip to Washington, D.C.--by herself! It was such a shock to me. How could a sickly, perhaps mildly retarded sister like mine take a trip to Washington alone?

Yet Sharon was perfectly capable of traveling to Washington or anywhere else--a capability I had a hard time seeing and spent time denying, in part, out of jealousy because I didn't have the guts to go to Washington on my own, but mostly because I had bought into my parents' view of my sister as one to be pitied and protected on account of her "problem."

"Don't tell anyone what happened; not your girlfriends or your teachers, nobody. People don't have to know what goes on here. It's nobody's business but ours."

"But what about all the people at church; they know, and you called the relatives and everybody. They already know, too."

"Shut up, Paula. You know what I mean, you big mouth. Just keep your trap shut."

But the "fainting spells" persisted.

Epilepsy. My sister has epilepsy. I can say that so easily as an adult, remote, removed. But even though I learned the name of her disease early, even though I often had to remind her to take the medication that controlled her convulsions, even though it was I, who, at eight or nine or ten had to remain with Sharon during one of these seizures, watch her, make sure she didn't fall off the bed, even though it was I who often had to run and search for a clean hanky to twist and knot and place between her teeth so that she wouldn't hurt her tongue because my parents were at work and it was "up to you, Paula, after all, you're her sister," still, my mother, through commands and scoldings, decided that this was not the word to use.

References to epilepsy became, "Well, you know. . .those fainting spells." Her disease became "Sharon's problem." And Sharon's problem, if that's what it was, became that of all of us. From the time of her first seizure, the family's attention was riveted on Sharon. Ours became a classic alcoholic family; all that was missing was the booze.

"Washington, why Washington?" I remember asking her as she showed me her tickets.

"Because I read in Glamour Magazine that that is where all of the eligible bachelors are, and I'm going there to find myself a husband."

"A husband? You? You've hardly even dated," I sneered.

"Who'd want to marry you, anyway?"

"I don't know," my sister sighed, ignoring the thinly veiled jealousy, the sarcasm that, from me toward her was incessant. "But I'll find someone. And when I do, I'm going to leave this family forever."

She went to Washington. Nothing "happened" except that Sharon met a lovely man who proposed to her during her week-long visit. She accepted. They married and began a life of army assignments in Germany, in Japan, in Alabama.

She got away.

And now that I had to call her, I didn't even have my only sibling's phone number. I had to ask a telephone operator for it.

Sharon's husband answered the phone.

"Steve, this is your sister-in-law--Paula. Is Sharon there?"

"Well, hi, Paula!" The surprise in his voice was unmistakable.

"Paula? Is that Paula?"

I could hear my sister in the background. I was astonished that she sounded so excited at the prospect of hearing from me. I felt nothing, because at that moment, it wasn't me on the phone calling my only sister, from whom I had been estranged for years, it was somebody else--a character in a play perhaps--and I was sitting in the darkened theater, remote from the actors on the stage, curious to see what would happen.

Then too, I reasoned, this was a business call about plans for our parents' Golden Wedding Anniversary. And if I remembered that, if I could keep it on a professional level, as if we were two business people who chanced to meet for a short while in an airport lounge, I could pull off the phone call without feeling sad or angry or so filled with resentment that it made me nauseous.

So we talked, and I was surpised to find that she sounded so happy. And she was funny. In some ways, Sharon seemed a lot like me.

We spoke tentatively about ourselves, our families. We had only seen each other's sons once; she had never met my daughter, her only niece. We had no idea what to do about our parents' anniversary, and so elected that Sharon would consult Aunt Jen, Mother's youngest sister, and get back to me.

That phone call was probably the hardest one I had ever made. I told no one about it, not even my kids, because there would have been questions--what's Aunt Sharon like? Can we meet her? Questions for which I had no answers. What was she like? I did not know; perhaps, I thought, I had never really known her at all.

About 9 o'clock one night just two weeks later, I had the chance to find out. I was standing on the front porch of a ranch-style house in Alabama and my sister was holding me in her arms. Five minutes later Ivan and Claire left with Sharon's boys, Steven and Matthew for fast food and movie rentals. They had suddenly found new cousins, good friends.

Sharon's husband moved quietly about the kitchen preparing a snack and brewing coffee as my sister and I sat down at the big table and opened the family photo album. We visited for hours with aunts, uncles, cousins. We found a photo of a boy in a striped shirt whom we had never met. He was standing with our mother's parents, looking awkwardly into the camera. He must be John, we decided, the uncle who was lost to us.

We felt the old question arise as we looked back 30 years at two little girls in party dresses proudly holding a white plush bear with red ears and penciled brows. And once again, the question arose: Could Mother really have burned poor Chedge? Could she really have done that to him? To us?

We poured over photos of Mother and Dad. Mother never smiled; she kept her arms folded and stood apart from the groups of friends and relatives who laughed and jostled each other in the photographs. Dad always looked ebullient in the early pictures, in his garden, with his parents, his wife, his children, his friends.

Then his smile slowly faded, disappearing somewhere among those black and white portraits that he loved to take as a newly-wed, a young father, a home owner, those snapshots that one day, simply stopped.

"Sharon," I began tentatively, "do you remember things, things that Dad used to do to us, and how Mother seemed to let him?"

Sharon looked at me for a long while.

"What do you mean, Paula? What kinds of things?"

"Well, French kissing, for example."

"I remember that, but that's all."

"Is it by choice that you don't remember?"

"It may be because I'm on so much medication, Paula. All I remember is the Frenching and one incident with the Good Humor man. But once I started having the seizures, Mother told Dad to stay away from me. And he did."

We did not say anything for awhile then, but simply sat together, turning the pages slowly as we had when we were little girls, sometimes stopping to peer at strange faces, to chuckle at an old-fashioned hairstyle, or to admire the beauty of Mother and our aunts.

Finally I looked at my sister and said, "Sharon, if I had not called you, would you have tried to contact me?"

She looked right at me.

"Never," she said.

"Isn't that sad? Being together like this feels so wonderful, so right. Yet it almost didn't happen. I wonder why."

Sharon closed the photo album, folded her hands across it, and leaned forward.

"I know why," she said. "Paula, after you got your Ph.D. Mother told me never to get in touch with you. She said you collected art and antiques and were a wealthy snob who wanted nothing to do with the commoners, that you only talked to other professors, and that if I tried calling you, you'd probably hang up on me. She'd say that every so often, over the years. And I believed her."

I turned and looked at Sharon hard. Was she lying? No. Why should she?

"Of course, there are two sides to this story, too, Sharon," I said, shaking my head. "I'd ask about you over the years, and it was always the same old thing, that you had become a born again Christian and wanted nothing to do with the riffraff of the world. Mother said that since the divorce you had thought of me as an adulterous whore and never wanted to see me again. And I believed her."

Sharon and I slipped our arms around each other. The truth had made us strong.

Chapter 33

Stop!

As a back-up to her therapy, Mary Elizabeth Hickman encouraged me to attend "anonymous" support group meetings in Bowling Green. She said it didn't matter which ones I went to; Alcoholics Anonymous, Narcotics Anonymous, Emotions Anonymous, and others would all serve the same purpose: to get me out of my office or apartment and with others who were struggling and supportive. At first it was nearly impossible for me to follow her instructions, so fraught with depression and loneliness was I. But whenever I forced myself to attend a meeting, I met kindly people whose stories and problems were far worse than mine; they made me get away from myself.

At the same time, the therapist loaned me *The Struggle for Intimacy*, by Janet Woititz, a remarkable book about adult children of alcoholics whose fragmented, chaotic, distrustful personalities belong to any of us from dysfunctional families, whether there was alcohol in them or not. That book had an astounding effect on me. For the first time I realized that I was not alone in my feelings or behavior.

My tears slowly released the years of pent-up anger and hurt, cleansing me. The Norpramine enabled me to think more clearly and function more easily: I actually completed several tasks every day--they no longer seemed insurmountable. Mary Elizabeth could see that I was becoming more stable emotionally, so one day, many months into therapy, she cautiously broached the problem of suicide by first emphasizing the positive changes she was seeing in me as the months passed. Then she said:

"Have you noticed that you seem to be dwelling less on the thought of killing yourself? When was the last time that you thought about it?"

I pondered for a moment. "Gosh, I guess I haven't thought about it in three or four days. I can't even remember now what set it off--oh, I know, I had a flat tire; that more or less topped off a pretty awful day. That's really amazing, isn't it, I mean, considering that suicide was all I thought about when I first started coming to see you?"

Mary Elizabeth smiled at me. "You feel proud of yourself, don't you Paula, that you had the courage to keep coming to Nashville to get help? Well, you should be proud. You are really healing."

"Right, thanks to you and Dr. Pate for believing in me."

"If you hadn't started believing in yourself, in your worth as a human being, you might not be here today. And you can get stronger still."

On impulse Mary Elizabeth gave me one of the warm hugs that she had had for me since the end of our first session--hugs that were difficult for me to accept at first, because I felt unworthy to receive them. The gesture still brought tears to my eyes. I looked at her, thinking how her outward loveliness, her blonde hair and blue eyes made bluer by her lavender dress, mirrored her inward beauty.

I looked at her for a minute and smiled. "O.K. I guess I'm ready to move ahead."

Mary Elizabeth sat back in her chair. "Great. You may think this next technique is just too simple to work for you, but I want you to start using it anyway. I want you to sit back, relax, and close your eyes. Good. Now I want you to picture a stop sign. I want you to see how bright the red is, and how big and white is each of the letters. Now I want you to look at the message on that sign and think about it until you can almost feel it. Okay? Now, every time you think about killing yourself, I want you to immediately envision that stop sign. Will you do that for me?"

I opened my eyes and nodded. But I had my doubts that something so easy would work.

The stop sign technique turned out to be the most challenging of Mary Elizabeth Hickman's assignments. It seemed so clear and simple. It didn't require anything in time or money; yet I could understand why she waited months to suggest it to me. That one simple method required that I change a lifetime of thought patterns.

The opportunity to try out the stop sign technique presented itself within the week. Three of my advisees in journalism had complained about my academic counseling. Why? Because I had advised each of them to change their major from print journalism to another area where they would be more certain to succeed. Each student clearly had potential, but it was not in a field where good writing skills are paramount, and each had refused to do rememdial work. I had offered to help the students in obtaining the appropriate academic and vocational testing, and to personally assist them in finding not only the academic department, but also the adviser within that department who would best serve their needs. I couldn't, in good conscience, sign them up for another term of our tough print journalism classes when they had already failed, or almost failed the ones they had attempted.

The upshot of my counseling was that I was reprimanded for suggesting they find new areas of study instead of encouraging them to, "do the best they could in print journalism. They may have to take a class over, but they can usually scrape by on the second or third try," I was told.

"And will they also be given second and third chances in such a competitive field where there are a hundred applicants for every job, or will we just let them scrape by in life?" I retorted. "Don't we have a moral obligation to these students?

"Shouldn't we care what happens to them, not only while they're in school, but once they've graduated?"

The exchange sent me into a tailspin. I questioned my principles, my conduct and my professional abilities, and somehow found myself wanting.

"I'm no good," I thought. "I'll just kill myself."

There was that automatic panacea--that shot of whiskey, that hit of cocaine. But I had been so proud of myself for not dwelling on suicide, that this time the thought jarred me. I went into my office, shut the door, sat down at my desk, closed my eyes and took a deep breath.

When I had envisioned the stop sign in Mary Elizabeth Hickman's office, it had been at the bottom of a country road by a pine-scented Northern Michigan forest. This time all I saw at first was blackness. I felt frightened-- maybe this was the answer, this death-like blackness. Suddenly, I saw dense grey smoke out of which emerged first an "S," then a "T," then an "O," and finally, the "P." I never did see the whole sign. But I did get the message. I kept spelling the word over and over and breathing deeply until the suicidal thought finally disappeared, and I remembered that I had other ways of working through my problems. I sat for a long time, strangely moved.

I knew the monster, suicide, would crouch and wait many times more, and I knew it would take a lot of practice to conjure up the stop sign quickly to hold the beast at bay. But today I could say, "So this is how it feels to confront the beast. And this is how it feels to win."

Chapter 34

The Phone Call

The phone rings, 11, 12 times. I hold my breath, sensing the pain as my mother tries to pick it up in her crippled hands, the fingers crisscrossed from 30 years of rheumatoid arthritis that has bent her body nearly in two.

"Hello?" Her voice is raspy, as if she has a cold.

"Hi, Mother, how are you?"

"Oh, it's you, Paula. Eeh! Same old thing. You know."

"Yes, I know, Mother. The pain. And do you have a cold, too?"

"Just some kind of congestion that's always there. I guess one day it will choke me, and then, goodbye! "

"Well, I'm sorry that you're having so much trouble, Mother. I wish there were something I could do for you. Where's Dad?"

"He's at the store. That's about the only place he goes anymore because he's burdened with taking care of me, poor thing! But he's been gone so long. Probably has himself some big-chested rich widow some place that he's fooling around with. Men! I'm telling you! I wish I had divorced him years ago. But, oh, well. At least he takes care of me. So how are you, Paula? What's new?"

"Oh, I'm fine, we all are. Ivan and Claire are getting so tall. And Ivan went out on a date Friday night--his second--with a real pretty girl who looks a lot like his sister."

"Did he dress up, or do kids go to dances now looking like bums?"

"Well, I don't think any of the kids dress like bums, but this was a casual dance. That's why he could go."

"You mean he doesn't know ballroom dancing, right, just that shake your ass stuff?"

"No, Mother, nobody waltzes at high school dances as far as I know. I think that ended back in the nineteenth century. No, I'm talking about clothes.

"When Ivan was so sick with the flu a few weeks ago and I stayed home to take care of him, I found him sitting on the couch looking at pictures in his wallet with this funny little smile on his face. I asked him if I could see the photos, and we looked at them together. They were all from these two dances at the high school last fall, and the kids looked so nice, all dressed up.

"When I asked him why he hadn't gone to the dances, he said it was because he didn't have the right kind of clothes to wear. I had bought him a nice sweater and a turtleneck, but I couldn't afford a blazer and dress slacks, which is what the boys wear. He's in men's sizes, and that means men's prices, you know.

"Our roof has been leaking for three months, and I've been saving for that. It's tough on the kids, but I think Ivan knows why our priorities have to be this way."

"How much do you need for the roof, Paula? Can I help?"

"Well, I've considered asking you for a loan from time to time, but no, I don't think so."

"But you need to get that fixed. If you don't, your house could really be damaged. The wood under the tar paper will rot, if it hasn't already, and your ceiling could fall in."

"Gosh, I didn't realize that. Well, the estimate I got was $500, which is a fortune to us. A loan would bring peace of mind, Mother. Thanks a lot."

"You're welcome! While I am able, let me help. That's what I'm here for. I'll get Dad to send you a check. You go ahead and make the appointment to have that work done. I'll get Dad to mail you a check tomorrow. Okay, my dear Paula?"

My eyes brimmed with tears. My parents had always been generous with money. "Okay, Mother. Thank you."

"Have you heard anything from your sister? She hardly ever calls us. Doesn't even send us cards, birthdays, Mother's Day, Father's Day. Oh, well, I guess she forgets. That problem she has makes people like her very absentminded, you know. But I always worry about her, poor thing. So sickly. I always pray for her."

"Mother, Sharon is not sickly, and she doesn't like you saying that about her. She's strong and healthy and she's made a good life for herself. She's doing really well in college, and she loves her classes. And she's got a wonderful husband and great sons. She is not sickly. She's busy. That's why she may forget."

"Still jealous of her, aren't you, Paula? And after all these years! You always did hate Sharon, always said things against her. Didn't I raise you to feel sorry for those who are less fortunate, and to help take care of them? You're as bad as you ever were, always thinking of your-- "

"What? What are you talking about? I love Sharon. I think she's great. I'm not talking against her, I'm explaining to you why she may not write!"

"Well, anyway, at least I love her. And I always like to hear from her, such as it is. She never complains. Never! Everything is always swell with her. She never complains, never calls here begging. At least I had one happy kid. I guess one out of two isn't so bad. Listen. I have to go now. My hand and arm are aching from holding this damn phone so long. Kiss your kids for me. I love you, Paula."

"Say 'hi' to Dad for me, Mother. And, uh, I love you, too."

Chapter 35

Yeast

My students at Western Kentucky University that semester had no idea what I looked like. I had suddenly developed sharp, stabbing pains in my right eye that could only be controlled by applying pressure. I taught those sixteen weeks with my left hand pressed firmly across my right eye.

What caused the pain? I consulted with two local doctors, who, despite several thorough examinations, were baffled by the malady. I finally consulted another specialist in the region, and he ordered a CAT scan. I had it done in Bowling Green, and met immediately after with a radiologist about the results.

"Here's your problem," the doctor said. "There's infection in the pituatary gland."

I felt hopeful; now that the source of four months' intense pain had been located, it could be treated. I took the X-rays to the physician out of town that afternoon, and as he examined the pictures, he talked to me.

"Just as I thought. There's nothing there. I've believed all along that we're either dealing with cluster-type migraine symptoms, or that--" he paused, turned around, and looked at me.

"You're divorced, aren't you? I always look for these kinds of non-specific complaints in women, especially. Why don't you take advantage of the holidays and get out and socialize a bit? Oh, and let me know if the pain worsens."

He was turning to leave the room when I told him to stop.

"What you just said to me is unforgiveable. Do you suggest to your male patients that a good lay will cure their problems, too? Friends have been telling me since I developed this infection in August of a physician in Kentucky who practices holistic medicine. Had I doctored with him in the first place, I would never have had to endure the humiliation you just put me through."

A week later, a friend drove me some three hours to the outskirts of Nicholasville, where Dr. Walter Stoll lives on eighty acres and practices medicine in a mobile home situated on a cliff. While I waited for the doctor to finish with another patient, I went outside to explore. I watched the brown water of the Kentucky River churning far below. It had been snowing off and on all day, and the wind hurled dry brown leaves at my feet. Icy flakes blistered my cheeks as I walked in the woods with the doctor's Airedale, Shakti.

"This is a strange and beautiful place for a healer to work," I thought to myself. "I know that he will help me."

There were other compelling reasons beyond his obvious love of nature that gave me confidence in this physician; one was the attitude of holistic physicians that patients are whole human beings and not just a series of treatable--or untreatable--parts. In contemporary practice, holistic physicians follow the wise example of great healers such as Edgar Cayce, who, in keeping with traditional healers everywhere, was as sensitive to an individual's mental and spiritual spheres as he was to the physical body. The goal of holistic practitioners is to find the root cause of a problem rather than simply to treat the symptoms. Thus, they are more likely to prescribe vitamin therapy, dietary changes and other life-transforming behaviors, such as meditation to reduce stress, than they are to dash off a series of prescriptions.

Yet holistic doctors are often targeted as medical quacks and are investigated much more frequently than traditional practitioners by medical licensing boards. Dr. Stoll had been in and out of the news, which made me hesitate to consult with him. And yet the persistent pain in my eye was very real--and thus far, untreated.

A telephone consultation prior to my appointment convinced me that I was on the right track. When I described to him the so far untreated infection, Dr. Stoll asked me a series of questions about depression, lethargy, frequency of upper respiratory infections and eating habits, then instructed me to bring along all of my medical records and to read *The Yeast Connection* by William G. Crook, M.D., before my appointment.

Even the early chapters of *The Yeast Connection* told me Dr. Stoll was on the right track. The author explains how Candida albicans, often the cause of infections of the skin, mucosa and vagina, can actually be the source of severe systemic diseases--including persistent infection and suicidal depression. I answered the Candida questionnaire in the book and scored more than 500 points on a test where 180 was considered a clear indication of yeast-related illness.

After a series of laboratory tests confirmed the presence of a massive yeast infection, Dr. Stoll prescribed and carefully monitored treatment with Nizarol and had me overhaul my diet. Candida grows on sugar in the blood stream. I had to eliminate all sugars, whether they were in something like a candy bar or cookie, or occurring naturally in honey, maple syrup or fruit. Trying to find sugar-free anything is next to impossible. I even had to limit my use of artificial sweeteners and give up caffeine. I had to cultivate an appetite for sugar-free, whole grain breads and cereals and for plain yogurt, which contains bacteria that help control candida in the digestive tract.

The diet was a difficult adjustment, but the results were amazing. My eye no longer hurt, I contracted no upper respiratory infection that spring, and the symptoms of depression that had plagued me, perhaps for a lifetime, lessened so remarkably that, with my psychiatrist's permission and continued supervision, I reduced my use of anti-depressant medication to short periods in the early fall and late winter as the seasons change. My fragmented life as a suicidally depressed person was mending, piece by piece. I was truly becoming whole.

Chapter 36

Drought

It was the year that the fire god walked, spreading his parched lips and breathing the hot breath that turned the creekbeds white with dust and baked the land dry as clean-picked bones.

Ivan and Claire went to visit their father early that summer, so I began freelancing for the Tennessean in Nashville as soon as classes at the university ended for the year, making frequent trips down I-65 to do research and conduct interviews for stories. In May, the temperatures were reaching August highs. There was no rain. The media carried so many stories about heat stroke that I began ignoring them.

One day as I was heading back about 3 p.m. from Nashville to Bowling Green, the air conditioning in my diesel engine car quit working. I opened both front windows, then got back on the road, trying to ignore the heat waves off the pavement and the ceaseless blasts of hot air. I reached for the iced tea I brought with me on these trips, but the ice had melted and the tea was hot.

My head was beginning to ache, and I saw black spots in front of my eyes. What were the symptoms of heat stroke? I couldn't remember. I started to panic when I passed a state patrol car with its lights flashing. The trooper was running to a parked car. The driver, a woman, was slumped over the steering wheel.

I tried to keep my thoughts clear as I looked for the Franklin, Kentucky exit that would take me to Bowling Green by way of 31-W.

Once on my favorite, two-lane highway, I began to feel better. There was less traffic, and the rolling hills and Victorian houses kept my mind off the light headedness I had been feeling on the interstate. I bought a Coke at the Frosty Freze, then drove slowly passed the Goodnight Memorial Library, and on into town beneath the canopy of trees.

Thirty minutes later I was back in Bowling Green, nauseated and feeling faint. If only I could make it home, where it would be cool. But as I pulled into my driveway, my heart sank. The blinds on the west-facing windows were up, and many of the old house's 19 windows stood open. The temperature was ninty-eight. The huge air conditioner sat on the floor of the garage, as it had all winter.

"I'll do it today like I said. Now quit nagging me. And toughen up. It's going to be a hell of a lot hotter than this, this summer. You'd better get used to it," the man I'd been dating for more than a year told me when I had asked him again to place the unit in the window.

"No," he said that morning, "I'm not too busy to do it. But if I get too busy, don't get any ideas about asking somebody else. I don't want any other guys coming around here." But finally, he'd promised to do it.

The heat in the house was ferocious. My only thought was to lie down before I fell down. I drank some water and managed to set up two fans in my bedroom. Then I blacked out.

Sometime later, I felt somebody shaking me, hard.

"Wake up, wake up. What's the matter with you? Sit up."

But I couldn't.

"I'm so hot, I'm so hot. I feel so sick," I said again and again.

I heard water running. Then he was pulling off my clothes.

"Go on, get in the tub."

I put my arms out, feeling for the walls to hold me up, then tripped and fell over my clothes. He grabbed me, shoved me ahead of him into the bathroom, and pushed me down in the tub.

"Why the hell did you come in here when it's so damn hot? Why didn't you go the mall or some place else that's air conditioned until the sun went down? For a university professor, you're pretty damned dumb."

I could hear him swearing as he climbed the stairs to Ivan and Claire's rooms. A short time later, he struggled past the bathroom door and into my bedroom, carrying a small window air conditioner that he installed and turned on.

"Wait fifteen minutes for that thing to start cooling before you get out of the tub," he said from the bathroom doorway. "Keep drinking water, and stay in your room with the door closed and you'll probably be o.k."

I could barely follow what he was saying.

"I feel so sick. Aren't you staying here?"

He snorted.

"You've got to be kidding. I'm going back to Rafferty's where it's cool."

"Back to Rafferty's?"

"Yeah. Me and my buddies knocked off early today. Too damned hot to work. Besides, we put in three, four good hours, so we figured we deserved a few beers. We've been, well, you know, keeping cool all afternoon."

"You're drinking again? But you promised--"

"Oh, shut up and cool down!" He paused for a moment. "Hey, could I borrow your car? Mine's on the fritz again, and I promised them I'd be back."

Once the bedroom cooled down, I could think more clearly. I refused to spend the summer in one room. I just had to get the big unit installed. I stood shakily and propped myself against the bed and an old wardrobe while I dressed. Then I moved cautiously through the dining room, across the kitchen, and through the laundry room to the back door. The evening air outside was cooler than the air within.

I leaned for a moment against the hackberry tree and looked across my long, wooded lot to the Alpha Gamma Rho fraternity house across the parking lot behind my property. Could I make it all that way? I had to.

When I got to the AGR house, I sat down on the back steps and waited. It wasn't too long before a pickup truck carrying two of Western Kentucky's agriculture majors pulled in. I told them I thought I had heat stroke and needed help with the air conditioner. Twenty minutes later, it was installed and cooling the house.

I was lying awake late that night when I heard my car's engine. The bedroom door slammed against the wall as my boyfriend rushed in and turned on the light.

"Where is he?" he shouted, looking about him.

"Where's who? What are you talking about? Turn the light off. It's hurting my eyes."

"Screw your eyes. Who put that unit in? Huh? Where is he?"

"You're drunk. Go on home and sleep it off."

Suddenly he grabbed my hair and jerked my head back.

"Look at me, God dammit. Who was over here?"

The muscles of his face jerked and his breath was sour from beer.

"Two AGRs. I asked for help and they came right over."

Now he was kneeling beside me, screaming, pinning my shoulders to the mattress.

"Didn't I say I'd help you? Didn't I? Didn't I?"

"Yeah, right. For two weeks. Some help. I take care of you when you're drunk or high, and you take care of me in the heat. We probably deserve each other, but I want you out of here. Go on, go home--and don't come back."

"Shut up, bitch, shut up! Or, I'll shut you up!"

His hands tightened around my throat. We struggled on the bed. I kicked him, hard, broke away, and staggered to the phone, but he was after me. The cord snapped as he tore the phone from the wall.

I grabbed my purse and ran wildly through the house to the car.

Chapter 37

Out of Control

About 6:30 the next night my two dogs and I walked eight blocks up Park Street to the old hospital on Reservoir Hill. I left Denzel, the coon hound, and Nelson, the English setter outside, and walked into the large room where 15 or so members of Women in Recovery sat in a circle on folding chairs, waiting for the meeting to begin. Many called each other by first names. Some laughed and joked. Others smiled pleasantly or lit cigarettes and watched the smoke blend with the early evening sun.

In a few minutes, the meeting began. We went around the circle, introducing ourselves:

"Hi. I'm Sherry," said a short, broad young woman with a pug nose and dark blue eyes. "I lost another three pounds this week." She clutched her hands over her head, prize-fighter style, and grinned while others clapped.

"My name is Leigh," a slender, dark haired woman wearing large gold hoop earrings said. "I've been clean six months. No drugs--and no men, either." Everyone laughed.

"Hi, you all, I'm Jolene, and I'm o.k. No booze, no complaints."

And so it went until each of us had spoken.

Sherry looked around the group and smiled. "Everyone seems to be doing o.k. tonight. Do we need to create an agenda? No? Doing great, girls! Nobody's having any problems? Nobody needs to share?"

Finally, I broke the silence. "I...I've never been to this group before," I began hesitantly. "But a friend told me to come because of what happened to me last night. She said you all would help me get back on track."

The women leaned forward. Some seemed to nod sympathetically as I described the drive from Nashville, my reaction to the heat, the lack of air conditioning, the realtionship, the attack. Then I sat back and wiped my eyes and nose with the Kleenex that had been passed to me from half way around the room.

"I guess that's all I have to say. Thank you for listening."

Leigh was the first to speak:

"Do you remember what it felt like when he was on top of you, screaming, with his hands around your throat? I mean, was it a kick? Didn't you love it?"

I was astounded at her insensitivity. But I had no chance no protest.

"Yeah. Didn't it feel good to you?" someone else asked.

"Wasn't it exactly what you wanted?"

I looked wildly around the circle. I saw comprehension. I saw disgust. I didn't see sympathy. What kind of friend would throw me into this pit of vipers?

"Paula, how long have you dated this man?" Sherry's voice was quiet.

"For about a year. Well, thirteen months."

She cleared her throat. "Do you do drugs? No? Alcohol? No? Then why would you hook up with someone who's hardcore?"

More tears welled in my eyes. I shrugged and looked down at my hands.

"I bet I know." It was Jolene who spoke. "Look at Paula. She's so soft and gentle like, I bet she just loves to help others, don't you, honey?"

At last, somebody in the group who understood.

"Paula, those wouldn't be your two hounds outside the door, would they, hon, the black and white one and the one with three legs?" Jolene asked.

"Denzel and Nelson. They came by my house one day so hungry that I fed them. And I never could find their owners. So I took them in."

Jolene pushed back her big red hair impatiently. "Have you had other boyfriends like this one? Ones who treated you poorly, I mean."

I nodded at Jolene. "Just about all of them have had problems. You know, loners...." I shrugged. "I've just always had all this love to give--if I love these men enough, and give enough of myself--then I can help them. You know, I can help them to get well."

I laughed a joyless laugh.

Sherry cleared her throat. "So you sort of rescue them, right?"

I looked at her and smiled wistfully. "Yeah. I sure try, anyway. I've always loved to help people. I was raised that way."

Sherry looked at me intently.

"And you came here looking for us to give you a hug to make you feel better and to pat you on the back and say what a great person you are for giving so much of yourself, for trying to rescue this guy, right?" Sherry asked between drags on her cigarette.

"Uh, I guess so," I said timidly.

She looked around the circle. "Should we do that girls?" she asked.

"Hell, no!" one woman called out.

"Are you kidding?" another sneered.

"Uh-huh, darling, we know all about those kinds of men. Do you know why we like them so much?" Leigh's voice suddenly took on a hard edge. "Because we're fucking fixers. Don't be selfish, that's not nice. Be considerate and thoughtful, like a good girl. Help this druggie, save that drunk. We're so goddamn busy controlling the life of every creep that stumbles across the doorstep that there's no time left to take care of ourselves. Stray dogs, stray men."

Leigh frowned down at her bright pink nails.

"Of course, there's no reason to fix ourselves because we're perfect, isn't that right, Paula?"

I could feel myself go red.

"No, no, " I stammered, "I'm not..."

"Well then, who the hell gave you the right to go off and play God? Paula can't rescue this man, or any other. The only one who can help

Paula is Paula, and until Paula is perfect, she can't go off and save anyone--anyone!"

I couldn't speak. I felt beaten up twice in twenty-four hours. Finally Sherry spoke. Her voice was gentle.

"Paula, we don't want to hurt you. Jesus, you've been hurt enough for one week. We're all just here to set you in the right direction, and do you know why we can?"

I silently shook my head.

"Because we've all been where you are, and we know it's hell. It's our job to pass on what we've learned. But it's up to you to use it."

Later, as I walked with my dogs down Park Street into the setting sun, I made a mental check list: change the locks, fix the phone--and unleash the strays.

Chapter 38

The Toad in the Garden

Sometime ago now, Ivan and Claire each asked for additional chores to earn money to buy me presents. On that birthday Sunday, Ivan gave me a hymnal and a silver chain with praying hands. Claire chose herbal teas, a gardener's journal and a fragrant purple hyacynth.

I held each of my dear children close and thanked them. My eyes filled as I watched them light the candles on the German chocolate cake they'd baked. I could see how my children loved me. But I couldn't feel a thing. I had been doing so well the whole winter, when suddenly, my beast was back. It had sunk its claws into me in early February. A month later its unbearable weight was still on my chest.

Monday was typical for early March. It was one of those gleaming, golden days filled with the radiance of pure light, a day when Winter becomes forgetful and stays at home, a day when Spring, shy maiden, breathes her warm sigh across the land and steps out, spreading her skirts in the fields and woods.

I could think of nothing but going into the garden. Perhaps if I spent the day out of doors with Nature, my beloved companion, my healer, then I would be better. But I began with a resentful and heavy heart. There was so much work to be done inside, so much more to do outdoors. I took up my spade and began hacking and thrusting and turning and churning the ice-laden spring soil, trying to transform it into something workable and fine.

I labored on, not in love, not in reverence for the world around me that was so very full of life, but in anger, in self reproach: I had a lot to do, but didn't everyone, and yet single parents have a double load. But I was on Spring Break from the University while Ivan and Claire were not, so that I had whole days entirely to myself. I shouldn't be depressed, I should be grateful! Yet I didn't feel grateful; did that make me bad? Hadn't the children given me a wonderful birthday? Could I not see how I was loved? Then why, why did I still feel so desperately depressed?

The black clods seemed so cold, so unyielding, so like me, dead in my impotent hands. I took up hunk after hunk, tearing them, smashing them, crumbling them, to make this earth do what I would have it do. Suddenly a clump began to move. I stood transfixed, hardly daring to breathe, watching the thing cupped in my hands. The hole from a roly-poly fell away, then an earth worm's narrow tunnel. This formless clod, this quaking, moving lump etched with the remnants of spring's final frost was taking on new form. Suddenly a tiny foot with spreading toes emerged, and then one plump, flexing leg.

I began holding the living clod tenderly, for here was life unfolding that I and my spade might well have destroyed. Gently, I crumbled bits and pieces of dirt away, periodically brushing and blowing, sometimes cupping my hands to warm the creature within, until finally, working slowly and patiently, I uncovered the hidden treasure: it was a warty toad, perhaps attracted by the rich compost and an ample supply of garden pests.

Exposed, the creature's heart beat wildly. The toad made a mad leap from my grasp, so I covered it with my hands and peeked at it, admiring the beauty and texture of its camouflage. Kneeling down, I put it back and crumbled the rich black soil over it. And as I knelt, I said a prayer of thanks for this toad, for this exquisite gift, a rich reward for my toil to beautify one small space.

And I asked forgiveness for my meanness, for my selfishness, for my narrowness, for my pride in ever pitying, ever questioning my fate. With difficulty, I also forgave myself. And then it came to me like light that each of us has beauty and our rightful job, a place in the order of things. To question, to resent, to attempt to control is unproductive, creates disease, and interrupts the flow in the natural order of things. But to live life--no matter how mean it might seem--willingly, lovingly, simply--is the path to wisdom and peace. I had found truth in a humble toad.

Chapter 39

The Voyage Inward

As I continued to make progress, to learn from the lessons that Life presented to me, and continued to work toward those days, weeks and months when I was free of depression because I felt so very good, I decided it was time for further self exploration. So, following the advice of Dr. Stoll, the holistic physician, I began to meditate, to voyage inward.

I read books by Native Americans, Eastern practitioners and those based on Edgar Cayce's teachings, joined a spiritual study group, discovered the best meditation posture for me, and learned how to keep my mind focused, how often and how long I should meditate, and about what I might expect to experience in this place of profound silence.

It felt strange at first to meditate, to sit in a chair with my spine straight, and my eyes closed when I had never felt comfortable closing them during prayer at church, to relax completely with my feet on the ground and my hands loosely opened, palms up, in my lap, to be absolutely still.

But I finally mastered the long, smooth cleansing breaths that I imagined as white light that I was drawing deeply into me from my genitals, through my stomach, my rib cage, my heart, my throat, my forehead, before releasing them through the crown of my head while exhaling just as smoothly and deeply. Later, I discovered it is best for me to meditate in a chair at my East-facing bedroom window that overlooks the Rose of Sharon growing wild there, or outside, sitting on the earth, spine straight against a tree in the pearl-grey light of dawn.

I had already struggled--and succeeded--in taking steps away from depression and suicide, steps that involved the emotional and physical realms. The more I meditated, the more I came to realize that total rebirth requires total recreation; I had been healed in mind, I had been healed in body; it was time to be healed in spirit.

I realized almost immediately that meditation seemed to lessen my depression. Sometimes I forced myself to meditate even when I felt too depressed to do so. I would go to the window, sit down, promise myself I only had to do this for five minutes, and then begin the deep breathing. By the time I was through, I often felt markedly better.

One day as I washed dishes, I analyzed why this was. For the very first time I understood that, when not singing or swimming or biking, I tend to be a shallow breather; the deep, cleansing breaths required at the beginning of each meditation oxygenate the blood. Could it be that as a shallow breather, there was inadequate oxygen going to my brain and too much carbon dioxide remaining in my blood, with the interplay between the two contributing to depression? I cannot say for certain. All I know is that whenever I think to breathe more deeply than I usually do, whether in or out of meditation, I feel instantly better, more alert, more energized, and far less depressed.

To enter into a meditative state I found it helpful to recite aloud the King James' version of the Twenty-Third Psalm, which, given its natural imagery, has always been my favorite Biblical passage. I read aloud from the White Eagle meditation books, and from Mary Strong's *Letters of the Scattered Brotherhood*.

I also began to repeat aloud, four times each, a series of aphorisms. "All things work together for good" is one. I found that each statement affirmed something of which I need to be forever mindful: that divine harmony and infinite wisdom are instantly available to those who seek; that love indeed overcomes all things; that truth and direction come to us when we are still; that the essence in each of us radiates sanctified light;

that the divine spark within unites us eternally with the everpresent world of Spirit.

The affirmations presented a major hurdle. I had never been a positive thinker. Now here I was, still sometimes deeply depressed, requiring of myself confident thoughts when I felt anything but. This exercise felt like Mary Elizabeth Hickman's STOP signs all over again. Why? Each required mental discipline, a word that had always made this rebel cringe because it carried with it a uniform and a smart salute. I had to set aside who I had been and literally create a new me. And yet, I reasoned, with myself, hadn't the STOP sign technique demanded that same mental rigor, and hadn't it made me feel much better, and far less suicidal?

And so I began to train myself, slowly, gently, day by day in the new ways, using the affirmations to mentally replace anger with acceptance, self-reproach with self-esteem, and fear with love, planting those positive seeds in the arid fields of my mind and heart, until, little by little, month by month, year by year, I became fresh and alive as I had never been before.

There is a great deal of truth in saying that we attract what we are. In those years of anger, frustration, self-debasement and emotional isolation, I knew many like myself. In fact, in those days, I seemed to seek people who had some element of danger about them. But as I began to meditate and to consciously ask for and work toward change, I began to attract others who, like myself, were seekers after peace and wisdom.

In meditation I have asked to be granted the ability to see clearly, to accept people as they are and not as I would have them be, and to always be especially grateful for the dark angels, who seem, in their behaviors and attitudes, to lay at our feet the most difficult lessons, yet who bring to us the opportunities for greatest growth.

I made the conscious decision to put violence out of my life forever. I broke my lifelong addiction to murder mysteries; I quietly ended all of the friendships I had with people who were sarcastic, intimidating, manipulative, or pessimistic, or whose sense of humor was cruel and debasing. I tried not to judge them as wrong, but as being at a place in their lives that was different from my own. I stopped watching hurtful films or television programs, including cartoons. And thus, little by little, I put thoughts of suicide aside.

Meditation has taught me to feel the difference between loneliness and solitude. Loneliness is an aspect of my uneasy beast, nervous, anxious, pacing, always in search of something, but never knowing what. Solitude is a profound sense of unity and harmony with everything there is; it places me at the center of things. I become a particle of divine energy in the eternal flow. Light and love came flooding in to cleanse the shadow from my soul.

I still sometimes unwittingly allow people and circumstances to pull me off my path. When I wake up and discover how far I've gone astray, I seek out sacred places to restore myself: Manitoulin Island in the blue waters of Lake Huron; Elizabeth's Dome in Mammoth Cave; a hiking trail in the Smokys; a boiling spring in the Missouri Ozarks; a major league baseball park; St. Joseph's Church in Bowling Green; any place, at sunset.

As I meditate this morning in the transparent light of day, I hear the drift of wind chimes from the porch. I carry the low, melodious music with me to that place where Truth and Spirit dwell, to that place where I find not death, but life, and, once again, peace.

Chapter 40

Ivan and Claire

The shrieks and whoops from the kitchen finally became too distracting.

"Hey, you guys," I called over my left shoulder, "I'm glad you think doing the dishes is so much fun, but could you please keep it down a little? I'm on deadline with this book, and I've just got to finish it before I go into the hospital."

Just as suddenly as the raucous noise behind me had started, it stopped. My eyes were on the computer screen, but my mind was now in the kitchen. I strained to hear my son and daughter's whispers.

"Mama," Claire wailed in a woeful way that always got my attention. "Mama, come here and see what Ivan did."

I sighed, pushed back my chair, and entered the kitchen. My children did not turn around. Soap bubble garlands dripped from the pale pink Pricilla curtains. Froth rose two feet high in the sink.

"One, two, three!" Claire counted rhythmically.

They snapped their fingers and turned on their heels.

"Surprise!" they shouted together.

Ivan's soccer-player haircut was a crown of suds. Thick bubble brows accented his bright blue eyes, and he sported a foaming mustache and goatee. Under Claire's smooth, dark page boy was a mask of white with two black eyes and pink lips.

"Ready, Ivan?" laughed Claire, swiftly loading her wooden spoon.

"Yep!"

I ducked, but not quickly enough. Claire catapulted suds into my face. The fluff Ivan maneuvered with his hands and his elbows settled like a cloud on my head.

"Oh, yeah?" I shouted. "This means war!"

Ten minutes later, we were collapsed against cupboards and appliances trying not to look at each other. Our stomachs could not bear more laughter. Finally, I crawled across the slippery floor, took the paper towels from the butcher's block, crawled back, and divvied up the roll.

Claire blotted the tiny bunches of lilacs on the antique wallpaper while Ivan and I wiped down the pale mauve walls and cupboard doors.

"I guess we needed this, huh?" I said after awhile.

"Yeah, the kitchen was pretty dirty," Ivan said, looking at his paper towels.

I chuckled. "No, Ive, not cleaning the kitchen, I meant our soap suds war. It broke down some of the tension we've all been under lately."

Ivan stood up, leaned back against the cabinet he'd been drying, and wiped his face in his sleeve. "So, Mama, are you worried?"

His dimples had disappeared, and his large eyes, which were usually turquoise, looked dark and troubled. He glanced at Claire, who had come to stand beside him at the counter.

"Worried? Let's see now. What have I got to be concerned about? The relationship? It was really wonderful while it lasted, and while I didn't end it, I can't spend the rest of my life dwelling on what might have been.

"Then, two weeks after the relationship ended, our car died. But I'm not worried about that, either. What can you expect after 160,000 miles? I've arranged to borrow money to have the engine rebuilt, and Bruce is a wonderful, honest mechanic. No worries there either, kids.

"Hmm. So what's left? Oh, yes. One week after the car died, the doctor discovered this tumor the size of a tennis ball."

I pointed vaguely to my belly button, then glanced up at my children. Ivan's braces glittered as he chewed on a fingernail. Claire's large black eyes were filling.

"When the doctor told me about the growth, I said it would be more appropriate to speak in terms of professional baseballs or soccer balls." Ivan and Claire did not laugh.

Ivan tapped his foot. "So, Mama, are you worried--about the tumor-- I mean?"

Suddenly Claire began to cry. "Stop calling it that, Ivan. It's not a tumor, it's a growth."

Ivan rolled his eyes. "That's what a growth is, Claire, it's a tumor. And if you don't like that word, it's because you're scared."

Claire began to cry harder. I pulled her to me and held her hard against my chest. With my other hand, I reached out and patted the shoulder of my son, whose fears often manifested as anger or impatience.

"I guess I worried about the tumor for just about five minutes after the doctor told me. Then I put it in perspective."

I shrugged and looked at each of my children. "What's always the worst thing about any problem? It's not knowing what you're dealing with, isn't it? So I'll have surgery, we'll give a name to whatever is in there, and then we'll treat it."

My son and daughter seemed unconvinced.

"O.K. You're waiting for the spiritual, philosophical explanation, right?"

Ivan and Claire grinned at each other. Claire hummed a note. "Hmm-a-maya-maya-maya," they sang. We all laughed. Then they looked at me.

"It's a gift."

"What's a gift?" asked Claire.

"The tumor. It's a gift of time, an opportunity to rest, to take stock of my life so far. It's a chance to see where I've been, and to decide where I'd like to go next, spiritually, professionally, even physically. I'm at a turning point in my life--I feel that so strongly. Now is the time to turn inward and take stock. Life has afforded me that chance. "

Now it was Claire who rolled her eyes. But Ivan ignored her.

"O.K., Mama. I know you don't like me to think negatively, but let's do a little hypthothetical. Oh, Great Spirit," he grinned and bowed, only half in jest. "Do not make this come true."

Then he straightened and turned to me: "What if you have cancer and you die, or the surgeon's knife slips, or something?"

I nodded. Those were possibilities. "There's money for each of you that's tied up in stocks and bonds. Please don't blow it all on cars and clothes. Spend it on education. Travel. Share some with others. I have two or three insurance policies; and since I have mortgage insurance, you guys would own the house, free and clear."

Ivan looked up in surprise. "You mean Claire and I could stay here?"

Turning to his sister he said, "I can drive now, so once Bruce fixes the car, I'll be able to take us places. And we know how to cook and do laundry and stuff. Gee, that's great. I can still play soccer for Bowling Green High next year."

Claire picked up where Ivan left off. "Yeah, and I'll be at the high school next year, so you won't have to drop me at the junior high, and I can look after the pets. Well, Smudge and Mouse, anyway." She scooped the black and white cat into her arms. The Siamese rubbed against her shins.

"That's fine. I don't mind taking care of Bentley." Ivan snapped his fingers. The golden retriever's 96 pounds were leaning heavily against me as I rubbed his ears. His tail banged the cupboard. He didn't budge.

I smiled at my children. "I'm so glad you've worked things out! There's just one small wrinkle--at 16 and 13, you're still too young to stay here by yourselves. If you want a guardian, you'll have to pick one for me to name in my will. Let me know what you decide to do."

As I left the kitchen to return to the computer and my writing, I could hear them drawing up a list. Sometime later, they came to me:

"Jurors, have you reached a decision?" I said in mock severity.

"We have, your honor."

I jumped up from the old walnut table. "Be right back," I called. I returned, my deep blue, velvet-trimmed doctoral robe swirling about me.

"O.K. Who's the lucky winner?"

"You are Mama," Ivan said. "Just have the operation and get better."

"Yeah, Mama," echoed Claire. "We like things just the way they are."

We all shook hands and hugged each other heartily.

"Thanks for the vote of confidence. Don't worry, I think I'll be back. These three weeks have really been tough for us, but it's times like these that strengthen us, that bring us closer together. We're surrounded by loving spirits. All we have to do is to let go our fears and to trust, believing always in the goodness of things. Besides, I've come to see life as the adventure it is."

I threw my hands up over my head and whirled around in my robe. "Notice, you guys, that I'm not depressed, and I don't want to kill myself! Life is like a wonderful book, or a movie that inspires and teaches; you can't stop reading, you can't stop watching. I want to know what happens next."

Ivan smiled down at me; Claire smiled up.

I hesitated, hating to spoil the glow of the moment. But it had to be said.

"In the minute particle of chance that my work for this particular lifetime will be finished with the book, let me leave you with a legacy that ultimately will be more important to each of you than houses or money:

"Love and honor the Earth, yourselves, and others. Do as you would be done by. Be kind and give help freely, but know the difference between enough and too much. Remember to accept love and assistance freely, too, for if you don't, you may be interfering with someone else's karma. Be objective and develop perspective. Cultivate curiosity and spend your lives in new places, learning new things. Maintain a balance among your physical, intellectual and spiritual lives. Keep material possessions in perspective, remembering, always, that less is more.

"Oh--and one more thing. If you have the opportunity to choose between cleaning your house and being outside, take a walk."

Chapter 41

January 9

I awoke early and went out to greet the new day. The trees and the grass were still heavy with dew, but the sun was shining, and the weather had softened; the grey skies and the chill winds that had borne the frequent, icy rains had passed. I knew that this was the day for which I had been waiting.

Returning to the house, I showered, put on the new dress and sandals and jewelry that I had purchased just a few days before, and took extra time with my makeup and hair.

I went down the hallway past the empty, silent rooms, made a brief telephone call, then drove out of the city, turning from the main highway onto the two-lane country road. The sky to the northeast was dark, smoldering. More rain, I thought, but no. Ashes were falling on the hood of the car, and a great flock of crows rose in a whorl above the burning brush, and above the crows, an eagle.

The man had driven his car from the main building, and was waiting by the wall.

"How can that be? How can there be wildfires? I've been here three weeks. We've had so much rain."

The man shrugged and began picking through a ring of keys.

"It's so dry here most of the time that even in a storm, if lightning strikes, everything burns. Florida's a tinderbox."

Finally, he found the right key, fitted it into a lock, and pulled open a small door. He turned one of the objects over, gave me a few instructions, then put both of them in cardboard boxes in my car. I followed his instructions to buy a small Phillips screwdriver. I focused my attention on this mission, and it carried me through the plumes of smoke, the shriek of birds, the chaos, the death that lay everywhere around me.

My mother had died in her sleep just before midnight on July 3, on the eve of Independence Day. Then, just five months later, on December 1, my sister Sharon was killed in an automobile accident on her way to work.

Ivan, Claire and I went down to Florida to spend the holidays with my dad, to share the loneliness, to ease the heart ache. In addition to having the three of us with him, what he wanted more than anything was a big, traditional Christmas dinner.

"You know what to fix, Paula. Cook everything just like we used to have it at home--turkey or chicken with homemade stuffing, sweet potatoes, mashed potates, gravy--the works. And use the good china and the silver, too."

The table was a groaning board lit with candles that filled everything with a wonderful light. I teased my dad, trying to bring a touch of merriment to the heartbroken holiday, fussed over him as I dished out his favorite casserole, then sat down across from Ivan, on the other side of Claire, and offered up a prayer of thanks.

The old mantle clock chimed among my final words: "And thank you..." One. "... most of all..." Two. "...for my dear dad..." Three. " Amen." Four.

And then my father died.

I placed the cardboard boxes on the back porch, then went in to the back bedroom to change clothes. As I crossed through the kitchen, a great wave of loneliness and sorrow passed through me, and I began to cry.

"I can't do this," I wept. "I can't do this."

"But you must," a voice from deep within me replied. "You alone must honor your parents' wishes, for there is nobody else."

I prayed for strength, dried my tears, then returned to the porch. Taking each urn from its box, I unscrewed the bottoms, and carefully, lovingly combined the ashes of my parents before separating them into two equal parts.

I carried half of them out into my father's gardens and looked about me for the place to begin. The trees in his little orchard were bowed, heavy with the lemons, grapefuit and oranges that he had not had time to pick. The purple plumbago and ivory gardenias were in full flower. Thirty amaryllis lilies were either budding, or just spent. Then my eye fell upon the bushes that my father had purchased on Christmas Eve.

"He knew--he knew that he, too, was going to die," I thought as I dug a trench, knelt, and gently placed the two white roses on either side of the one with the deep red blooms. Then, praying and singing softly in a ceremony that I hoped was befitting of the memories of my father, my mother, and my sister, I mingled the ashes of my parents with the sweet, rich earth and watered it with my tears.

It took nearly the whole afternoon to complete the ceremony in the garden. At dusk I drove south across the bridge into Punta Gorda, then headed west. Finally I parked the car and began walking through the tall sea grasses, sometimes stumbling in the soft sand dunes, pressing the precious cargo against my chest. At last I came to a place where cyprus trees and sea grapes nestled in a tiny cove that was warmed by the setting sun.

Once again, I knelt, sang and prayed.

I cast a handful of ashes on the softly rolling waters.

"I love you both."

Another handful.

"The trials in my life have been to strengthen me."

Another handful.

"You have been my teachers, Dark Angels. I am grateful for every lesson, for each has strengthened me."

Another handful.

"May you be at rest with Sharon in the Creator's embrace."

I cast the last of my parents' ashes into the flowing waters of the Peace River, and with love, acceptance, and understanding, I let them go, I let them go.

Chapter 42

Valleys and Summits

I was home alone, writing, when the morning sounds at the window distracted me. There they were, all five of them, and their mother; six blue jays at the feeder, in the rose of Sharon, toppling to the ground, trying their young wings, crying for food, calling their messages to the wind.

Suddenly, I heard a voice so clear, so close that I turned. Someone stood behind me in the empty house. But no one was there. When I sat down, I heard the voice again: "Each ascent to the summit begins in a valley. Consider the beauty of valleys."

What did it mean? I sat, thinking for a long time about the valleys which I had crossed, out of which I'd ascended alone: Nearly a lifetime of sexual, physical and emotional violence that I had vowed with every fiber of my being not to pass on to my children, and not to repeat in my own life; the triple valleys of a home, a marriage, and a job all gone at once, buried in an avalanche of pain; perfectionism and pridefulness that would not let me ask for help; the inability to love and forgive self, and thus, others; the loss of my mother, my sister, my father, all within five months' time; the healing of the addiction to suicide.

Then I considered the slow ascent that had carried me to my beloved Kentucky, to friends who are like family, and ultimately, to physical, emotional and spiritual rebirth, and to understanding, acceptance and forgiveness. And as I began to comprehend the wisdom in those words, I felt the wings of peace enfold me.

I stand forever on the pinnacle of a new life. I hear the wonder of the silence. I watch the golden light of dawn and see the snow that melts in the new day, cascading down the mountainside, feeding the waterfalls, the freshets, greening the grasses, rushing over the cress, inspiring the wildflowers to bloom.

I contemplate the path that I have just traveled, with its stony places and smooth, with the boulders that nearly forced me to give up. And I watch those coming after me in the universal flow. To one I shout encouragement, to another I give my staff, for the final steps to the summit can be as trying as the first.

Then I turn toward the light and shade my eyes to glimpse what lies ahead. I see another valley. How beautiful it is.

A portion of
the sale of each book...

...will be donated to a program of traditional healing at Wikwemikong First Nations Unceded Reserve, Manitoulin Island, Ontario, Canda.